Suddenly

SUCCESSFUL

*How Behavioral Optometry
Helps You Overcome
Learning, Health And
Behavior Problems*

**Hazel Richmond Dawkins
Dr. Ellis Edelman
Dr. Constantine Forkiotis**

Optometric Extension Program

Printed in the United States of America
Published by the Optometric Extension Program Foundation, Inc.
2912 South Daimler Street, Suite 100
Santa Ana, CA 92705-5811

Editor: Marcia Castaneda
Managing Editor: Sally Marshall Corngold
Illustrator: Kyo Takahashi

First Edition, 1991

Library of Congress Cataloging-in-Publication-Data
Dawkins, Hazel H. Richmond.
    [1st ed]
    Suddenly successful : how behavioral optometry helps you over-
come learning, health, and behavior problems / Hazel Richmond
Dawkins, Ellis Edelman, Constantine Forkiotis.
      p.   cm.
    Includes bibliographical references and index.
    ISBN 0-943599-14-8 :
    1. Behavioral optometry--Popular works. I. Edelman, Ellis S.,
1924- . II Forkiotis, Constantine, 1923- . III. Title.
RE960.D38 1991
617.7--dc20   91-9807
                                              CIP

Dedications

To all those in behavioral optometry, practitioners and patients, who have shared so much with me, particularly Dick Apell and John Streff, but above all, to my wife Roslyn, my children Marcia, Bobby and Chuck and my grandchildren Joanna, Jennifer, Lon, Scott and Jordan.

Ellis S. Edelman

To my optometrist, Amiel W. Francke, to Dorothy (Pat), my able-bodied assistant, without whom my office would not run and my public service work could not be carried out, and to my daughter Carol.

Constantine J. Forkiotis

This is for Colin and the Dawkins clan, my mother Emily, and Alexandra.

Hazel Richmond Dawkins

TABLE OF CONTENTS

Foreword

Decades of research proves without doubt that the quality of the eye's functioning, more precisely, the functioning of the vision system, has an effect on the brain and involves the autonomic nervous system. Those optometrists knowledgeable in the complete care of the vision system can correct inadequate visual performance through the use of optometric vision therapy.

A very high percentage of my young patients who are diagnosed attention deficit disorder do not use their eyes well to converge and track. Most adults who were "learning disabled children" reveal the same visual defects.

I have been treating patients suffering from the attention deficit disorder since the 1970s and have referred most of them for examination and visual training to optometrists who practice optometric vision therapy. This therapy is valuable in the treatment of learning-disabled adults, because learning-disabled children untreated grow up to be learning-disabled adults. Age is not a factor in the development of visual performance skills; such skills can be developed at any age.

Over the many years, I have sent patients to Dr. Forkiotis and to other behavioral optometrists. An examination of a learning-disabled child without a consultation and treatment by a behavioral optometrist is an incomplete examination and treatment.

This book is an authoritative publication which identifies visual problems in understandable language. While it is important reading for parents of children with learning or behavior problems and for adults with more subtle problems, it is also informative to practitioners who work with such youngsters or adults. It makes an invaluable addition to libraries everywhere.

Allan Cott, M.D., New York City.

Authors' Preface

This book was first commissioned by Dodd, Mead, one of America's oldest publishers. The editors there were very enthusiastic about the predecessor to this book, the little paperback, *The Suddenly Successful Student, A Guide to Learning and Behavior Problems,* which had been published in 1986. The Dodd, Mead editors approved wholeheartedly of the outline and sample pages and the first chapters of the manuscript of this book. When the material was half written, startling and sad news came: Dodd, Mead was on the verge of bankruptcy. Ultimately, this venerable publishing house was closed.

This left us with a manuscript but without a publisher. For a while, a British publisher was interested. He faded from the scene more silently than fog. By now, over two years had passed. We were anxious to see people reading the book. Into the breach came the Optometric Extension Program Foundation. Their Board of Directors voted to support the publication of the book and finally we were off and running.

Collaborations such as the one that produced this book are rare. The trio whose names are on the title page, Ellis S. Edelman, O.D., Constantine J. Forkiotis, O.D., and Hazel Richmond Dawkins, worked closely and in harmony. They were fortunate to be able to draw on the expertise and support of optometrists across the United States and around the world.

Busy practitioners returned phone calls, sent articles, case histories and other literature and encouraged the work as it progressed. If one wanted to present the research from places such as the Gesell Institute of Human Development and the colleges of optometry, as well as the accomplishments that occur daily with this therapy, one would need an encyclopedia. The collaborators settled for this book.

Drs. Edelman and Forkiotis have specialized in optometric vision therapy for decades, painstakingly gathering the knowledge presented here. To this, writer Hazel Richmond

Dawkins has brought personal experience. When she was seven, she had an operation to "straighten" an in-turning eye. Within months, the eye was turning out. For the next forty years, Hazel was blind in that eye. Legally blind is 20/200, she measured 20/400. During those years, Hazel was told by general practitioners of eye care in England, France, Switzerland and America that nothing could be done for this blindness although the eye was "healthy."

Imagine then, her amazement when she was referred to Dr. Edelman and learned that her "blindness" was the result of the brain shutting down input from that eye because it didn't fuse with the input from her other eye. She discovered there was a distinct possibility she could learn to straighten her eye, without surgery, and perhaps recover some of the lost sight and vision. In the months of optometric vision therapy that followed, the changes hoped for did materialize.

In rapid succession, Hazel's husband, Colin, and four of their five children consulted with Dr. Edelman and were helped to an extraordinary degree. At this point, Hazel enlisted the collaboration of Drs. Edelman and Forkiotis. The result was the paperback, *The Suddenly Successful Student, A Guide to Learning & Behavior Problems*. The trio then decided that the subject deserved several more books. This is the second.

Many willingly offered their help and their support in the years since the collaboration began, for which the authors thank them. Special thanks go to Drs. Richard Apell, Beth Ballinger, Beth Bazin, Nathan Flax, Elliott Forrest, Amiel Francke, David Friedel, Lynn Helerstein, Stan Kaseno, Charles Margach, Robert Sanet, John Streff, Irwin Suchoff, and Baxter Swartwout and Glen Swartwout. An enthusiastic appreciation also goes to our reviewers, Edna Jones and Drs. Martin Birnbaum, Allan Cott, Dorothea Linley, Tom Rose, and Morris Wessel. The help of Bob Williams and the staff at OEP has been invaluable.

Fact Sheet

Behavioral (also described as functional or developmental) Optometry is a rapidly growing therapy in the field of optometry.

Roughly 30 percent of the individuals in any school, college or office have difficulties with learning and work that have nothing to do with their natural intelligence. Their problem is with their vision.

Youngsters with vision problems are often labeled slow learner, problem child, learning disabled, dyslexic and delinquent.

Most vision imbalances are triggered or aggravated by stress, or the visual demands of work or computer use.

Sight and vision are not the same, there is a critical difference between them: Sight is the ability of the eyes to focus, one of many different skills that make up vision. When skills such as converging, fixation and teaming integrate efficiently with the brain's visual cortex so you understand what you see, the result is vision.

Sight is the ability to "see," to look at an object and have it in focus. When we use our vision, the brain organizes the information "seen" and gives it meaning, often by relating it to our other senses and past experience. Vision is the ability to understand what is seen.

Vision develops in a sequence of predictable stages. Therefore, it is trainable.

Vision problems may trigger or aggravate health, learning or behavior problems. When behavioral optometry brings balance to vision, often the health, learning or behavior problems may be helped and will respond to traditional therapies such as remedial education or counselling which might not have been effective before optometric vision therapy.

The concepts, practices and lens use of this optometric therapy are different from general optometry and ophthalmology. In general, most lenses prescribed are "compensating." Behavioral optometry uses lenses in ways that are "remedial," "developmental" and "preventive."

Remedial lenses are for a specific problem, such as an inability to sustain focusing, until that ability is adequate.

Developmental lenses are to support and nurture an immature vision system while helping it develop normally and cope with visual stress.

Preventive lenses are to prevent a problem in the vision system from starting in those individuals diagnosed "at risk."

The ability to see and correctly interpret what is seen does not appear automatically at birth. It develops during the first twelve years of life and is shaped by health, your experiences and the environment.

Optometrists -- The O.D. degree stands for Doctor of Optometry. It is earned after a minimum of seven years of college and graduate education. Appendix I compares typical professional programs in optometry, dentistry and medicine. Optometry's areas of specialization range from contact lenses to pediatric vision. One of the most innovative is vision therapy, for which postdoctoral training needed.

General Optometrists offer routine eye health care and refraction (the clinical measurement of the eye to determine the need for lenses). Their extensive education has prepared general optometrists to detect not only ocular diseases but signs of certain health problems such as hypertension, diabetes and arteriosclerosis.

Behavioral (developmental or functional) Optometrists practice vision therapy, sometimes in addition to general optometry, sometimes exclusively. In contrast to general optometrists and ophthalmologists, who usually believe that visual problems stem from random or genetic biological variations, behavioralists believe that visual problems are also triggered by environmental factors which may be developmental or stress-induced.

Ophthalmologists are doctors of medicine (M.D.) whose post-graduate training is in diseases of the eye.

Opticians are technicians who produce and/or dispense the optical lenses, glasses or other equipment prescribed by optometrists and ophthalmologists.

Optometric vision therapy works on the visual perceptual system (the eye, oculomotor muscles and pathways, the optic nerve and optic tract and that part of the brain used in vision processing). Warps or imbalances at any point in this complex system will lead to faulty processing of visual information. This in turn may trigger a host of behavior, learning, work and health problems. This therapy is often able to:

- prevent or modify vision imbalances such as myopia (nearsightedness) and astigmatism;

- develop the visual abilities and skills needed to achieve at school, work and sports;

- enhance visual functioning;

- reduce or eliminate chromic health problems, including travel sickness, bed wetting, light sensitivity, migraines, tension, teeth-grinding, muscle pain, depression, alcoholism and schizophrenia.

Age is not a deterrent to the benefits of optometric vision therapy. Infants of two months can be helped, adults in their seventies can benefit.

Health insurance companies such as Aetna Life & Casualty Company and Blue Cross/Blue Shield have plans that cover optometric vision therapy -- and have done for years.

About the Authors

Hazel Richmond Dawkins is a veteran editor-writer whose career began in London's Fleet Street Newspaper World and has since taken her to Paris, Geneva and New York City. She has worked for major publishers including Harper & Row and Columbia University Press.

Ellis S. Edelman, O.D., received his doctorate in Optometry from the Pennsylvania College of Optometry and is a graduate of the Gesell Institute's postdoctoral course in behavioral optometry. An Associate of the College of Vision Development and the Optometric Extension Program Foundation, Dr. Edelman specializes in optometric vision care at Newtown Square, Pennsylvania.

Constantine Forkiotis, O.D., was a classmate of Dr. Edelman at both the Pennsylvania College of Optometry and the Gesell Institute. A Fellow of the American Academy of Optometry and the College of Vision Development, Dr. Forkiotis is active in many organizations, including the Connecticut State Board of Education. In private practice, Dr. Forkiotis specializes in optometric vision care in Fairfield, Connecticut.

The Connecticut State Police have used the behavioral optometric vision programs Dr. Forkiotis developed for them since 1970. A consultant for the U.S. Department of Transportation Research Office and the National Health Traffic Safety Administration for drug-testing detection and the National Standardized Behavioral Sobriety tests, Dr. Forkiotis was invited by the State of Iowa to present an Expert Witness Course to Police Training Officers, State Prosecuting Attorneys, County Attorneys and Behavioral Optometrists in 1985.

Kyo Takahashi, an internationally known artist, is also an author who illustrates his own work. A Vice President and Senior Art Director at Lintas: Campbell-Ewald of Detroit, Mr. Takahashi was formerly with J. Walter Thompson in New York.

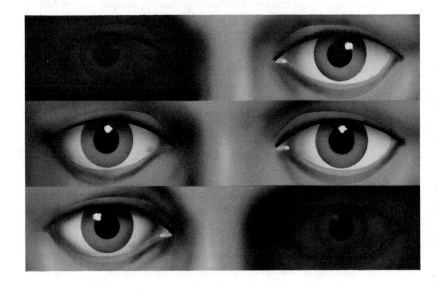

This art represents one of the most important abilities of the vision system: teaming. If your teaming is inadequate, your perception of what is going on around you is not accurate.

Chapter 1

A Road Patrol with Vision

The December night was dark. The Connecticut countryside was peaceful. One of the two officers sitting in the front of the patrol car spoke to the man in the back. "You know, it doesn't matter how often you're out on special patrol, you get tense. From the time you first see a driver acting in a suspicious way to the time you confront them, there's a big question mark. You hope it's someone who's had a few too many drinks, but there's always the chance it is a criminal, or a loony tune or someone who's flaming mad at the whole world."

The man in the back seat of the patrol car, Dr. Constantine Forkiotis, nodded. He knew about the stress involved in police work. He'd written papers on it, after spending years working directly with police officers. He was about to speak when the sound of a car going into a skid broke the calm of the New England countryside. Tires protesting in a scream, a Mustang snarled round the corner, sliding across the road. The sporty car lurched to a stop inches short of a telephone pole.

"Are they lucky," murmured one of the police. "Now, their luck runs out. Why won't I be surprised if the driver fails the nystagmus test?"

Driving Under The Influence

Hours later, their tour over, the special patrol for DUI (Driving Under the Influence) was headed back to the station. The mood of the three men in the police car was one of exhilaration. Gone was the tenseness. In its place was satisfaction at having done their work well, at knowing the courts would back them up with convictions for the charges of driving "under the influence, whether alcohol or drugs."

Until now, such cases had often been thrown out of court for lack of evidence. The night's road check had netted a good bag of "suspiciously erratic" drivers. It was safe to say these drivers would be convicted on the basis of having flunked the latest and strongest test to date, the one for nystagmoid oscillation, or an uncontrolled, erratic eye movement. A lay person might say the eyes were not moving smoothly but were twitching or jerking.

Experts such as Dr. Constantine Forkiotis, a behavioral optometrist, are aiding police across the United States learn to test "suspicious" drivers for nystagmoid oscillation. This test is helping keep the roads in America safe from people driving while under the influence of alcohol or drugs. The test is based on the concepts of behavioral optometry.

What Does the Test Show?

"Doc, if you have time when we get back to the station, we have a new officer who's really interested in the nystagmus test. She's just been transferred here and hasn't been to any of your lectures yet. One of her sister's kids was killed by a drunk driver, who got away with it. I told her I thought you'd probably show the test to her yourself, so she can see it at the hands of a pro." The officer driving the car smiled at Dr. Forkiotis. He'd known the optometrist long enough to be sure he'd do it if at all possible.

"You know I'll be glad to talk to her or anyone else," came the reply. Once they were back at the station, a small crowd of police officers gathered when the news spread that the optometrist was going to show the new officer the nystagmoid oscillation test. Dr. Forkiotis held up a pencil level with the police officer's face."Can you see this clearly?" Dr. Forkiotis asked."Yes, just fine," came the answer. "Good. Now please keep your eyes on it as I move it from side to side. I want you to follow the path of the pencil from left to right and back again. Are you ready to start?" "Sure." Obediently, the woman's eyes followed the pencil as Dr. Forkiotis moved it slowly in front of her several times. "Well, Officer," Dr. Forkiotis said, "I'm glad to say that your eyes are tracking smoothly. No nystagmoid oscillation."

"One question, Doctor. What would you see if I did have a nystagmoid oscillation?" "What we're looking for is a variation, an instability from the normal smooth eye movement as you move your eyes and follow the path of the object, in this case a pencil, as it travels from side to side. If someone is 'under the influence,' one eye will lose its ability to move in coordination with the other. That's the oscillation. This is an involuntary movement, you can't learn to control it or fake it while under the influence either of drugs or drink. You just can't move the eyes smoothly in synchronization with each other while 'high.'"

"This stands up in court?" asked the new police officer. "It's really accepted?" "Ah, yes," Dr. Forkiotis replied. "Sometime, I'll tell you about my trip to Iowa. My court appearance there was pivotal to the acceptance of this test. We were challenged by a group of experts. They lost. They just hadn't done the right research. They had no idea there's a wealth of scientific support for the behavioral optometry which is the basis for this test."

"Weren't you in California, too, doctor?" questioned the desk sergeant."Yes, with the Los Angeles Police Department, under the auspices of the US Department of Transportation Research Office. I did appear for the State of Maryland as an expert on alcohol gaze nystagmus, which is what the test is also called. I was in court in New Hampshire, too. Successfully. You'll learn more about the practical applications of behavioral optometry because my work at the Academy includes checking that each officer's vision is as good as it can be."

What Is Optometric Vision Therapy?

This book is about a health care that is of supreme importance to your well being: optometric vision therapy. A specialty in the field of optometry, and labeled behavioral, it offers a remarkable approach to resolving learning, health and behavior problems which are vision-related. The therapy's range is astonishing. So astonishing that after prize-winning screenwriter Alvin Sargent completed work with behavioral optometrist Dr. Moses Albalas of Los Angeles, Sargent went to the Walt Disney Company and recommended that a documentary on behavioral optometry be made. He did this because he found that his optometric vision therapy with Dr. Albalas had changed his perceptions. The studio listened to Sargent, who has received academy awards for his scripts, which include "Ordinary People," "Julia," and "Paper Moon." "The Mind's Eye: The Experience of Learning," directed by Terri Straus, came out in 1986 and is featured regularly on the Disney channel.

Optometric vision therapy is of value to people who are highly motivated (like Alvin Sargent and a roll call of professional athletes such as members of the New York Yankees, Chicago Black Hawks, San Francisco 49ers, Dallas Cowboys and US Olympic athletes). It also is of value to people, young and old who struggle with all manner of unresolved learning, health and behavior difficulties. Optometric vision therapy is able to:

- Prevent or modify nearsightedness (myopia) and astigmatism

- Develop the visual abilities and skills needed to achieve at school, work and play

- Reduce or eliminate chronic health problems,
  including travel sickness, bed-wetting, headaches,
  migraines, tension, teeth-grinding, light sensitivity,
  muscle pain, chronic depression, schizophrenia,
  juvenile delinquency and alcoholism

Regretfully, optometric vision therapy will not rid us of all such problems. This is because this health care is effective when problems are related to the way your vision system works.

Our eyes are the external receptors for the intricate vision system. One of the most important abilities of that system is teaming. The art on the first page shows what happens when there is faulty teaming--sometimes you do not have the full picture of what is going on all around you. This means that when reading, working at a computer or on a back hoe, driving a car, walking across a room or playing sports, you may not always have accurate perceptions of the situation, even though you believe you do. Faulty teaming, all visual problems, are subtle, hidden processes. The results are not.

You may have excellent eyesight, perhaps the proverbial 20/20. Yet vision problems may be present, and they will interfere with your ability to learn and play efficiently and comfortably. This is because over 70 percent of what you perceive, remember and understand depends on the efficiency of your vision system. The following definition of vision is the result of a collaboration between Dr. Robert Sanet, a behavioral optometrist in Lemon Grove, California, and his staff:

Vision encompasses the ability to track, focus and coordinate the eyes together as a team. Visual discrimination, form perception, visual memory and the integration of visual information with other sensory systems are all included in the complex act of vision.

Optometric vision therapy works on the visual perceptual system, which includes the eye, the oculomotor muscles and pathways, the optic nerve and the optic tract, as well as that part of the brain (the occipital cortext and the areas of the cerebral cortex--parietal and temporal lobes) used in vision processing. Warps or imbalances at any point in this complex system may lead to a host of behavior, learning, work and health problems. Other factors, such as heredity, our parents' health and stress also play influential roles in the vision system's development and functioning. Pollster Louis Harris says in his book *Inside America* that 89 percent of all adult Americans report they experience high levels of stress daily.

Although we may not recognize the symptoms, the stress of learning or working is frequently a major disruption to the efficiency of the vision system. When the vision system is in good balance, the harmony in your body makes it easy to learn, behave, work or play efficiently. Your health may also benefit because of the intimate connection between the vision system and the hormonal system.

A succinct description of this therapy comes from Nathan Flax, M.S., O.D., a noted author in the field of behavioral optometry. A professor at the State University of New York College of Optometry for many years, Dr. Flax has a private practice in Garden City, New York.

> *Optometric vision therapy is an organized therapeutic regimen designed to treat neuromuscular, neurophysiological and neurosensory conditions that interfere with vision function.*

More Than Eye Care

Dr. Flax explains that optometric vision therapy must be distinguished from routine eye care, which is required by everyone and involves infrequent visits to eye care practitioners. "Vision therapy, on the other hand, is not required by all people. It often involves extended care to treat a diagnosed condition."

In his book, *Vision Enhancement Training*, practitioner Dr.

Albert L. Shankman of Norwalk, Connecticut, explains his experience has led him to the following definition:

Vision takes place in the mind.. It is the product of how one's mind perceives time, space and causation. These perceptions are the basis of one's habits. One's habits have a direct relationship to the development of one's personality. Any modification in the perception of time, space or causation will result in a modification of vision and personality.

He adds that this definition has helped him understand why the same procedures do not result in the same benefits for all patients.

The American Optometric Association estimated in the 1990s that 1 in 5 of the elementary schoolchildren in the United States had vision imbalances that hobble their learning and development. The incidence of severe vision dysfunction among the general population is estimated at 9 percent. This climbs sharply to some 66 percent for severe problems in those with clearly diagnosable psychiatric disorders.

The "How" Of Optometric Vision Therapy

Several options are offered with this therapy:

1. Lenses or prism use

2. Optometric vision training

3. Lens or prism use combined with the optometric vision therapy

These three options distinguish this field from the practice of other professionals in eye care. One option is to do nothing, for there is no doubt that many people who have vision imbalances do manage to "cope," handling their lives as best they can. However, it is usually at a high price, because their health, efficiency and personal relationships often suffer as a result of the problems created by untreated vision imbalances.

Your Work, Your Results

Practitioners of optometric vision therapy are women and men with truly unique professional training. But it is you the patient who does the work and who benefits from the results. Certainly, the expertise of the behavioral optometrist guides the patient and prescribes the lenses, prisms and procedures used, but the patient brings motivation and gives time and effort.The overall purpose of optometric vision therapy is to create a change in the way you perceive and integrate information received through the vision system--and that is 70 percent of the information we handle each day. The purpose of the therapy is to influence the entire system rather than to improve just one aspect of vision, such as clarity of sight.

If you want to learn tennis or baseball or if you are training for a new job, learning experiences are usually partnerships: the pupil and the coach. Optometric vision therapy is no different. This powerful therapy can help you make trans-formations in your perception of your life because it offers you the tools to change and improve your life.

Do You See Anybody Here That You Know?

Jimmy   A third grader who still can't read, even though he is obviously bright, even though the school system is clearly a good one.

Debra   A seventh grader, labeled "lazy, disruptive and un-cooperative," despite tests which show that she has a high potential.

Sam   A teenager who has become surly and withdrawn, dropping out from school and life. He was not that way in his early years.

Hope   A wife and mother of three children. She has never been able to catch a ball; gets violently travel sick;

has blinding headaches and although Hope loves sewing, she just can't do close work for long.

Manfred   A middle-aged man who is intelligent and skilled at his work, but he falls apart when given responsibility and promotion.

Luci   The daughter of a President of the United States. A school failure. Subject to severe headaches and nausea after reading and studying.

These are real people who had real problems. Their case histories or others like them are discussed in this book. Their problems are not uncommon. In fact, they are all too common in today's pressured world. In each case, physicians, therapists, teachers, families and friends had proposed all kinds of reasons for the problems: The patients were emotionally disturbed, they were brain damaged, they weren't quite right, they were angry at the world. In many cases, the individuals involved came to believe these unflattering descriptions of themselves and suffered greatly from feelings of failure and lack of self-esteem. This borders on the tragic because their problems all derived from vision imbalances, despite the amazing fact that their sight was good

---

Sight and Vision are not the same, there is a critical difference between them: Sight is the ability of the eyes to focus, one of many different skills that make up vision. When skills such as converging, fixation and teaming integrate efficiently with the brain's visual cortex so you understand what you see, the result is vision. Sight is the ability to "see," to look at an object and have it in focus. When we use our vision, the brain organizes the information "seen" and gives it meaning, often by relating it to our other senses and past experience. Vision is the ability to understand what is seen. Vision develops in a sequence of predictable stages. Therefore, it is trainable.

Vision imbalances triggered their difficulties with their learning and in some cases laid the foundation for behavior, learning and health problems. Until they were examined by optometrists who practiced optometric vision therapy, their vision imbalances went undiagnosed and unhelped.

Problems Very Close to Hand

Many of us, young and old, have problems with our vision, problems that in turn often cause physical discomfort, distortions in posture, the pain of migraine and, inevitably, difficulties with learning and behavior.

Unfortunately, few of us realize when our vision systems are not functioning properly. The signals are hard to connect with the causes. Also, most vision problems can be detected only by special optometric tests. These tests are best performed by an optometrist who practices optometric vision therapy. Optometry, like other health disciplines, has many areas of specialization besides behavioral optometry. They include contact lens work, low vision, sports vision, pediatric and geriatric care.

The practice of optometric vision therapy takes aptitude and years of postdoctoral work. Few ophthalmologists or general practitioners in optometry have been exposed to the necessary intensive education and training. The concepts of the therapy are based on the scientific truth that you may have decent sight but vision is possible only when all the systems work together harmoniously.

Over the past decades, this therapy has had a considerable impact on the lives of many. By the mid-1980s, its concepts were applied nationally in the United States by the police, with the nystagmus test for detecting driving while under the influence of alcohol or drugs (the test measures erratic eye movements). The federally funded studies of delinquents who were wards of the Juvenile Court in San Bernardino have shown how this therapy radically alters the face of juvenile delinquency. Yet sadly, the therapy is little known by the general public or, to be candid, by many members of the health care community. Those who do know of it, however, endorse the therapy with enthusiasm.

This is the first consumers' guide to optometric vision therapy. From the historic background of this therapy to insurance coverage, to information about practitioners, clinics, colleges and institutions around the world, you will also find case histories to help you understand the depth and range of this unusual health care. This guide discusses all aspects of a health care that proves 20/20 eye care is not enough for those with behavior, learning or health problems triggered by vision imbalances. The answer is optometric vision therapy.

Juvenile Delinquency Affects Us All

Judge Ander of the Juvenile Court listened carefully as the case details were presented. The teenager's record listed three previous convictions for serious offenses against the county. Glancing over the file in front of her, the judge saw that the accused, "Jimmy," had turned sixteen on July 15, just two months before.

"Your Honor, in view of the offender's past record and the severity of the offense, we're asking for a minimum sentence of two years with the California Youth Authority."

The judge nodded. She had reviewed the case load before court convened and noted that Jimmy had committed robbery with violence for the second time. She'd also read that the youngster had repeated a grade in elementary school and had received special education courses, tutoring and counselling. The boy had shown a serious pattern of learning problems early. Yet he'd had the full battery of attention from the school district. Was there any way to reach this young offender? The judge made her decision. After she had pronounced sentence, she added a qualification in a final effort to offer Jimmy help.

"Let Doctor Kaseno see this young man at the Juvenile Hall Vision Clinic." The probation officer nodded in agreement.

Jimmy shrugged indifferently. He'd been through it all. Nothing worked. Why did they keep on trying?

A few weeks later, Jimmy was sitting in Dr. Kaseno's office, stolidly enduring an exam. It occurred to him it was different from others he'd had in the past. The teenager had been surprised to discover that this doctor was an optometrist.

"We do special therapy for your eyes and your vision," Dr. Kaseno told him. "My eyes are just fine," Jimmy said defensively. "You're right," came the reply. "You have good, healthy eyes and 20/20 sight. But we can help you improve the way your vision system works."

After Jimmy had gone, Dr. Kaseno went over the exam results with the technician who would be giving the teenager therapy from the program custom-designed for him.

"Jimmy has visual difficulty reading. After a page or two, the print blurs and runs together. His eyes start to tear, he skips lines. He says it's been that way as long as he can remember. "The IQ test shows a 90, but at this stage, we can't use that as any accurate indication. The boy's hand-eye coordination is so poor, we're hardly able to measure intelligence accurately. The IQ test is done with paper and pencil and Jimmy has extremely poor visual abilities. His eye tracking, alignment and focusing are erratic and visual processing skills [the ability to read and understand the material] are virtually nil."

Dr. Kaseno passed the file over to his assistant.

"You'll find a program outlined for Jimmy. He'll start next week, for twenty-four therapy sessions. Two a week for twelve weeks. Our approach here is a little different from the usual practice, where an hour is usually the recommended time. We give therapy only in half hour sessions. These youngsters are too stressed, visually, to handle more than that. They literally don't have the visual stamina or attention span to handle their schoolwork."

One month later, Jimmy had made progress, good progress.

He was much more comfortable reading, because the therapy had helped improve the quality of his eye movements. Two months later, Jimmy was reporting proudly on his improvement in school. His teachers confirmed his claims. They were delighted but not too surprised, because for the past seven years Dr. Kaseno and his staff had upset all previous figures, blazing a phenomenal track record with juvenile delinquents, helping youngsters no one else had been able to help.

Jimmy was known to the teachers at the San Bernardino Juvenile Hall. Altogether, he'd already spent several years in and out of the hall, courtesy of the county. Now, for the first time, Jimmy was learning in the special juvenile hall school. There was little doubt that undetected visual problems had hindered him in the past. Now that the visual impediments to his learning were being removed, he was making true progress.

When Jimmy had completed his three months of optometric vision therapy, he was retested for visual efficiency, IQ and grade level. The improvements were significant. His eye movements were smooth and controlled. Focusing changes occurred efficiently and his visual processing skills (reading and comprehension), had grown and expanded. He was now at an 8.3 grade level for reading, compared with the grade 5 level at which he'd initially measured. His IQ was now 94, an increase of 4 points.

Dr. Kaseno had not taught Jimmy reading. Dr. Kaseno had worked with the teenager's vision system. In a September 1985 article in *Academic Therapy*, "The Visual Anatomy of the Juvenile Delinquent," Dr. Kaseno commented, "What was very interesting to us was that this increase in reading skill was achieved without any change in the academic program at the juvenile hall." Jimmy himself was proud of the changes in his classroom work, but he was really enthusiastic about the way he'd improved at sports. "I can see the players on the court, they don't blur," he reported to the vision clinic staff. "I'm shooting baskets easily and mixing the shots now."

Jimmy is one of hundreds of juvenile delinquents treated by the vision clinic staff in a federally funded project in southern California. The results are inescapable: this therapy is critical in reversing delinquency.

"Optometric vision therapy is not the only factor in the plight of the juvenile delinquent by far--just a critical missing link," says Dr. Kaseno. A 1989 report to the legislature of the State of California noted: "The date available, nevertheless, indicated that the recidivism (the percentage of wards arrested or who violated court orders) for Regional Youth Educational Facility wards, after six months in the community, is 16 percent compared to 45 percent for a carefully constructed comparison group."

A Successful Track Record With Delinquents

Spring 1987 in sunny California. Fullerton, to be exact. Fifty power brokers from across America--a mayor, staff people from legislators' offices, psychologists, community administrators--listen intently as an imposing panel of nonoptometrists present their accounts of the results of optometric vision therapy on juvenile delinquents.

The seminar is sponsored by the Southern California College of Optometry (SCCO), the College of Optometrists in Vision Development (COVD) and the Optometric Extension Program Foundation (OEP). The audience is here because they asked to be invited. In the months before this symposium was convened, they had caught the media's message about the people-saving, money-saving results of optometric intervention with juvenile delinquents. This therapy was the only one that had not previously been made available to the young offenders. These influential people had seen and heard Dr. Stanley Kaseno, director of optometry at San Bernardino Juvenile Hall, on the MacNeil/Lehrer News Hour, in a four-part news series on Channel 9 in Los Angeles and on a twelve-minute documentary by the Canadian Broadcasting Company.

Now they took notes as people prominent in the field of

juvenile delinquency spoke. Among those they heard were Thomas Hefter, M.D., chief medical officer of the California Youth Authority in Ventura, W. Russel Johnson, Ph.D., staff psychologist at the University of California-Irvine Medical Center and Judge Lawrence Kapiloff of the California Superior Court. They also heard from some of the behavioral optometrists present, including Michael Rouse, M.S. Ed., O.D., Associate Professor and Chief of Vision Therapy Services at SCCO, and Dr. Kaseno.

The Bottom Line

Behavior that breaks our customs and laws tears the fabric of our society. No one wants to live with the havoc of violence. In an attempt to remedy whatever wrongs have caused juveniles to erupt into antisocial behavior, we offer young offenders a host of remedial services and therapies. Custodial care costs the government of the United State staggering amounts daily. A way has not yet been found to lower these figures.

The success rate for reducing the level of recidivism in the United States is not high. The norm for rearrest is 50 to 60 percent. The costs have been high, however you count them-- the loss to society of potentially valuable members, the victim's personal loss, the financial sums needed to incarcerate and care for juvenile offenders.

The drawing card in the use of behavioral optometry for juvenile delinquents in the California system is the success rate. When you couple Dr. Kaseno's results with the fact that this therapy was the only therapy not previously made available to juvenile offenders, it's irresistible economics.

"We find an absolute correlation between vision disorders, reading disabilities and juvenile delinquency," says Dr. Kaseno. "Most forms of intervention aren't working, but no program works well without the youngster's ability to learn and think problematically. I'm working with murderers, rapists and burglars as well as other offenders. The hardest for the courts to place in treatment facilities or foster homes are those who commit the most heinous crimes. These individuals, often described as incorrigible, get the most from our therapy program because they stay the longest in the facility. Generally, the average stay is fifteen days and we do not treat short-term inmates. At the vision clinic, we're only contracted to work with delinquents with long sentences."

A Seven-year, Federally Funded Project

Dr. Kaseno began the program in San Bernardino's county prison system in 1980. The project first had federal funds, then was continued under the jurisdiction of the county probation department. A six year follow-up study of over 500 juveniles showed the re-arrest rate went from 45 percent to 16 percent. Findings from the programs supported earlier studies made by optometrists David Dzik of Tennessee, Roger T. Dowis of Colorado and Joel Zaba of Virginia.

How did optometric vision therapy help where other therapies involving huge sums of taxpayers' money had failed? The juvenile delinquents seen by Dr. Kaseno had such massive vision imbalances that they were rarely able to benefit from other therapies until optometric vision therapy brought some sort of balance to their visual systems. When you give remedial education, tutoring or counseling to youngsters with vision imbalances, it's like trying to drive your car with the brakes on. You won't get too far. Would you try to nail down floorboards without a hammer? As this federally funded study has shown, learning problems and antisocial behavior change after optometric vision therapy. Once some harmony and balance exists in the vision system, then the youngsters can begin to benefit from traditional education.

Dr. Kaseno's strategy for working with delinquents is carefully planned. Perhaps the most important factor is that individual programs are charted for each youth once the youngsters have been given the first visual analysis and screening. Therapy involves the use of lenses, prisms and a wide variety of procedures: moving disks with pictures, walking rails (you shuffle, wobble or edge your way across a 4 x 4 on the floor, kid's stuff until you add the special lenses or prisms), balance boards and trampolines are some of the devices."The heart of the therapy is to improve visual tracking, focusing and processing skills and train the five senses to work in harmony," said Dr. Kaseno. "Most of these youngsters have poor focusing ability and need to learn to control their eye movements. Most could not read for more than five to ten minutes at a time without discomfort. During the early days of the study, support had to be won from professionals with other backgrounds.

"Psychologists, teachers, counselors and others were skeptical at first and reluctant to cooperate, but now that the results have been seen, they are routinely referring youngsters for therapy."

Dr. Kaseno recommended 396 evaluations and performed 250. Of these, 60 percent had accommodative infacility (difficulty focusing), 59 percent failed tests of eye pursuit movements (an object like a pencil is moved back and forth, from left to right in front of you; normally, your eyes will follow, or track, smoothly). A high number, 83 percent, had symptoms of poor attention span, poor comprehension, headaches and other clues that often indicate visual dysfunction.

"I couldn't have started my work without the original work of Dr. Dzik, who initiated this type of study in the late 1940s and early1950s. He was the ultimate pioneer. He motivated others like Drs. Dowis and Zaba and myself," says Dr. Kaseno.

When he began applying for federal, state, county and private grants in 1974, Dr. Kaseno failed to attract any interest. Four applications and six years later, the son of a county official received optometric vision therapy with one of Dr. Kaseno's colleagues, a behavioral optometrist who retired shortly thereafter. The youngster benefited enormously from the therapy. This prompted his father, who was chairman of the county board of supervisors, to contact Dr. Kaseno with the question:

Will this therapy be any help to the rapidly swelling population of juvenile delinquents?

The efforts of this official were critical in the final quest for high-level support of the federal grant application. Now a well-placed bureaucrat had firsthand, intimate knowledge of how the therapy worked and the types of results that could be anticipated. The circle was complete.

But Will the Horse Drink?

When optometric vision therapy is deemed a failure, it is often because the patient just wasn't motivated enough to wear the lenses or practice the procedures. How, then, did Dr. Kaseno persuade the juveniles?

"We had to use psychology in order to sell them on the idea. Generally, since the budget is restricted, one is tempted to buy basic frames. We asked the youngsters to select what they wanted. Naturally, they wanted whatever was the fashion. We found we could usually order reasonably priced copies, and because it was what they wanted, they'd wear them. Later, we found that in the wards it was a new form of status symbol to have the prescription tinted glasses.

"Gradually, the youngsters themselves would send in their buddies. They were able to recognize how the therapy had helped them. Just about every delinquent here wants a way out. They've had so many therapies tried on them before, they have a sense of failure. At first, they approached us with negative attitudes. Why would this work any more than anything else had? That changed."

The rearrest level was not the only change. The reading level zoomed an average of three grades, from 5 to 8.5 grade level; the mean average IQ rating went from 90 to 94. All of this after a minimum of 12 vision therapy sessions (two half-hour sessions each week) and lens use for that period of time. The maximum therapy length was 24 sessions. Perhaps one of the most valuable factors in this equation is the change in personal esteem and confidence.

In the early 1980s, it cost the county of San Bernardino $30,000 annually to incarcerate and care for each offender. Society loses more than that, though, when we lose whatever contributions these youngsters might have made in their communities. The victims lose, and again, we all suffer. Clearly, if it's possible to change the picture of delinquency, this will benefit all. The therapy's intervention, at a cost of approximately $600 for each youngster, has changed the way the delinquents perceive their lives and themselves. It has changed their ability to handle their schoolwork. The majority have not returned to prison. That saves more than tax dollars. Society can anticipate rewards beyond financial values. Consider the question inherent in the study: Why wait until youngsters are reduced to juvenile delinquency?

Chapter 2

Those Early Years--An Unusual History

Most people wonder why they haven't heard about optometric vision therapy, particularly when they're told it's valuable in so many different circumstances and has been available for decades. Others are puzzled when their physicians either do not know about the therapy or oppose it. When you read about the complex background, it becomes easier to understand the situation.

The history of optometric vision therapy is the rare story of a health practice that began in one camp and ended up in another, in a radically different form. European ophthalmologists, the medical practitioners who specialize in diseases of the eye, were responsible for the nineteenth-century development of vision therapy's distant cousin, orthoptics. By the twentieth century, orthoptics had served as the launching pad for American optometry to develop its innovative vision therapy.

A Space Age Transformation

A word of warning here. Any attempt to compare orthoptics with optometric vision therapy is like comparing the Wright Brothers' aircraft with the space shuttle. Both are forms of transportation, but they are light years apart in concepts and results. So it is with orthoptics and optometric vision therapy. The concepts, practices and results are radically different.

The intricate connection between vision and behavior has been observed throughout the centuries and documented by scientists and philosophers. Your body, your background and your lifestyle all affect your vision system. In turn, the vision system influences behavior and health.

The surgeon to Socrates, Alcmaeon, concluded from his dissection of animals and humans that the eyes were connected to the brain by certain pathways. He theorized that visual sensations met and integrated there with memory and thought. Prescience! The 1981 Nobel Prize for Medicine went to three researchers for work which linked brain processes and occipital lobe neuron growth to visual perception and understanding later in life.

A good history of vision therapy is by optometrist Leonard J. Press, Chief of Vision Training Service and Associate Professor at the State College of Optometry of the State University of New York (SUNY). The history is in Appendix VIII of "Vision Therapy and Insurance: A Position Statement," a 1986 publication by SUNY. Readers interested in looking at this well-documented history might telephone their local optometrists for a copy; members of the College of Optometrists in Vision Development are likely to have this publication. If you're fortunate to live near one of the fifteen colleges of optometry in America, ask your local library to arrange an interlibrary loan for you or a local optometrist to borrow the position statement from the college for you.

Unique Qualifications

Two factors have played a large part in optometry's involvement with this innovative therapy:

1. Lens and prism use, an inseparable part of vision therapy. American optometrists have a unique knowledge of physiological optics. Lens and prism use are combined with a specialized analysis of the vision system.

2. The American optometrists who pioneered the practice of this therapy recognized that drug use would interfere with the examination of the vision system by changing the patient's physiology. Although by the 1990s, state after state in America had begun licensing optometrists to use drugs for diagnostic and therapeutic purposes, the development of optometric vision therapy was structured without use of drugs or surgery. Undoubtedly, this situation may change. The Wright Brothers did not conceive of space age technology because it was in the future.

Dr. Nancy Torgerson of Seattle, Washington, and Dr. Tirsa Quinones of New Haven, Connecticut, explain that they and many of their colleagues have taken the rigorous licensing exams because of their desire to understand the effects of drugs on the human system.

"This knowledge increases my ability to work more efficiently with ophthalmologists and other M.D.s, who prescribe medication for patients referred to me," says Dr. Quinones. "All optometrists have this type of training during their college years, but the number of drugs has increased and so much more is known about their effect and interaction one with another. Much will depend on the type of practice an optometrist has, but I felt it would enhance my ability to offer the best type of optometric vision therapy possible."

The Precursor: Orthoptics

Vision therapy as it is practiced in the 1990s stems from basic optometric techniques in use since the 1950s, although the origins go back to the 1850s. Today, this therapy is used to correct or help the effects of a wide range of visual and perceptual disorders. The historical roots of vision therapy spring from the nineteenth-century practice of orthoptics, which literally means 'straightening of the visual axes."

A French ophthalmologist, Dr. E. Javal, is considered the father of orthoptics. His personal interest in this type of therapy as an alternative to eye muscle surgery came from the poor results of operations on his father and sister. Actually, he called the surgery "a massacre."

Dr. Press says that "although first suggested by du Bois-Reymond [a French ophthalmologist] in 1852 and MacKenzie [a British ophthalmologist] in 1854, it was Javal who formulated many of the procedures still in use today in the discipline known as orthoptics."

British ophthalmologist Dr. Priestly Smith visited Javal in France in 1896 and brought back his methods to England. In 1903, Dr. Claud Worth, a prominent British ophthalmologist published the first edition of his classic text on squint (strabismus). In it, he wrote:

These rhythmic exercises do not increase the power of the ocular muscles any more than voice training increases the power of the pharyngeal muscles, but they often improve the power of dynamic convergence [the act of turning the eyes inward to look at a near object], by teaching the nervous apparatus to respond more readily to the will.

Almost a century later, that point is still blurred. It is one of the main causes for the lack of understanding about optometric vision therapy. This health care is not "eye exercises," or "muscle gymnastics." Rather, the therapy is training of neurological pathways.

While the practice of orthoptics was growing rapidly in England and France at the turn of the twentieth century, it was comparatively unrefined in the United States. A 1904 book authored by Dr. Valk, a surgeon at the Manhattan Eye and Ear

Hospital, reflected significant growth in American ophthalmologic thought. Dr. Valk considered orthoptic treatment preferable before consideration was given to surgery. He explained that the treatment worked on the individual as a whole: "The ocular muscles are not the reins to drive a horse or simply to move the eyeballs in, out, up and down, but these beautiful anatomical structures of the eye are controlled and adjusted according to the laws of nature and also controlled by the human being behind it all that must influence them in many ways."

In that paragraph we see the start of the thesis which Dr. Forrest developed so eloquently in his 1987 book, *Stress and Vision,* that our mental states, beliefs, biases and attitudes are highly involved in creating what we are and what we become, visually and otherwise.

A Quantum Leap

1904 was also the year that two British ophthalmologists authored a provocative essay on childhood squint. Optometrist Dr. Press suggests this "may have been the seed of behavioral vision training. Drs. Browne and Stevenson stated that the "blackboard and chalk formed the most valuable means of combining the exercises needed by squinters...." Their treatment of strabismus included bimanual drawing on the chalkboard; they also trained visual perception in this way.

A comprehensive text on stereoscopic eye exercises authored by Dr. David Wells, an ophthalmologist at Boston University Medical School, undoubtedly marks the beginning of orthoptics in America. A warning note is sounded when Dr. Wells notes in his preface that many ophthalmologists ignored the importance of binocular problems (simultaneous use of the two eyes in the act of vision) unless the patient had strabismus (one eye pointing in a different direction from the other). He also noted that binocular vision was an intricate psychic faculty and "its inefficiency could result in an inability to fix one's mind on study and reading."

This statement is as true today as it was when written in 1912.

Indeed, it is pivotal to the concepts of behavioral optometry. Dr. Wells initiated a careful treatment program which was soon incorporated into the practice of many ophthalmologists around America.

It might seem that by now, orthoptics would be firmly established as a beneficial health therapy. A text published in 1927 by Dr. 0. Wilkinson, a Washington ophthalmologist, is voluble in its praise of orthoptics for a variety of vision functions. Predictably, next came the professional organizations. In 1937, the British Orthoptic Society was formed, a year later the American Orthoptic Council was established. A few years later, however, the situation had changed drastically.

The Fork In the Path

Apparently, ophthalmologists in the United States were becoming less satisfied with the results of orthoptics. Several reasons for this were given in a 1945 article on American methods in the British *Orthoptic Journal*, which commented that American ophthalmologists "made the mistake of expecting the already overworked secretary or office nurse to supervise this treatment--and usually these good ladies do not even have an elementary knowledge of orthoptics." This would not seem too difficult a situation to remedy, but the article went on to make a vital point:

However, the approach to the whole idea of orthoptic treatment is that it is more or less a passive treatment for strengthening ocular muscles instead of re-educating the cerebral process. Naturally, very little if any success results.

Dr. Press notes in his history that this situation in America in the 1940s "led to the evolution of current orthoptic practice, wherein knowledgeable orthoptists are certified and based in institutional or specialty settings."

Optometry Develops Vision Therapy

In the 1920s, A. M. Skeffington, O.D., began to seek different approaches to lens use and concepts in American optometric practice. In their book *Eye Power*, Ann and Townsend Hoopes explain that to find answers for his questions, Dr. Skeffington travelled widely and incessantly, "challenging the conventional wisdom of a conventional profession with a fine cutting edge and continually examining and reexamining his own positions."

The 1920s and 1930s were decades of unusual collaborative clinical and research work. Optometrists, ophthalmologists and visual scientists developed the field of visual perception at the Dartmouth Eye Institute in Hanover, New Hampshire. The contribution of this era was significant, for it heralded the principle that perceptual changes are brought about by ophthalmic lenses, a concept integral to optometric vision therapy.

Sightseers and Visionaries

In 1928, when the Optometric Extension Program, now the Optometric Extension Program Foundation (OEP), was founded by E. B. Alexander, O.D., Dr. Skeffington became OEP's first Educational Director and the mainspring of the foundation for forty years. The first organization to develop a wide variety of continuing education courses for optometrists and to publish pamphlets for the public, OEP is today international in scope, its several thousand members spread around the world.

Dr. Skeffington's approach was creative, involving authorities from other disciplines, among them Samuel Renshaw, Ph.D., an experimental psychologist at Ohio State University. Dr. Renshaw's lab work was responsible for the theory of vision, which anticipated by ten years the cybernetic theory of perception, as well as other concepts vital to the development of optometric vision therapy. Another giant whose resources were tapped was John Paul Naffe, M.D., then considered the world's authority on skin and its function.

Professor N. Kaphart, an industrial psychologist and associate of Dr. Alfred A. Strauss, one of the first to explore the performance of "brain-injured" children, was also a player on Skeffington's team. Perhaps one of the most distinguished contributors was Dr. Darell Boyd Harmon, a renaissance man noted for expertise in such diverse fields as pediatrics, kinesiology, architecture, lighting, engineering, pedagogy, penology, human performance and vision. As Dr. Forrest wrote, "Though he was not an optometrist, his scope of knowledge was such that it left a strong imprint on behavioral optometry."

Visionaries like Dr. Skeffington, his wife M. J. Skeffington, M.D. (an ophthalmologist), and optometrists Alexander, Brock, Eberl, Getman, McCoy, McQuarrie and MacDonald, through their scientific collaboration and experimentation over the decades from the 1930s, synthesized knowledge from many fields. They absorbed and built on basic principles. One was the theory of Piaget, Swiss psychologist and biologist. Piaget reasoned that a child's cognitive and intellectual development proceeds in stages that always follow the same sequential order.

Another major force was the important work on child development by Arnold Gesell, M.D., and his staff at what became the Gesell Institute of Human Development. Dr. Gesell, Dr. Skeffington and many others collaborated for many years. Their work is discussed in the section Vision and Behavior: the Unbreakable Link.

By considering vision and its functioning in the light of a diverse range of principles, the early American optometrists were able to build a solid foundation for behavioral optometry. Gradually, the work of pioneers from many fields established the foundation for the development of optometric vision therapy. A record of the therapy's growth exists in the many publications of OEP, beginning in 1928 with what is generally regarded as a landmark text by optometrist R. H. Peckham. Valuable writings by Drs. George Crow and Harry Fuog were published by OEP in 1937 and 1938. These works established a clinical model for the rehabilitation of visual disorders other than strabismus and amblyopia, the areas on which ophthalmology had concentrated.

By the 1950s, optometric vision therapy had evolved from theories to programs which typically integrated visual, auditory, kinesthetic and tactile functions to help patients reach the peak of their performance. The concepts of the unique lens and prism use had also been developed through the original approaches of leaders such as Dr. Amiel Francke, Dr. Richard Apell and Dr. John Streff. More and more, optometrists became involved in early childhood programs and school vision screenings as well as educational and industrial consultations. Preventive and enhancement programs were offered.

Now a science, branches of specialization such as sports vision began to be formed. Optometric vision therapy became part of the curricula of many of the colleges of optometry, some of which also had clinics for this specialization. Up to the 1950s, OEP had offered the only postgraduate clinical associateship, through a series of lectures, regional and national seminars and local study groups throughout America. The Gesell Institute in Connecticut began its postgraduate fellowship programs in the 1950s. The College of Optometrists in Vision Development was formed in 1971 as a certifying body for Fellows who engage primarily in optometric vision therapy. In 1973, the American Academy of Optometry established a Diplomate Program through its section on Binocular Vision and Perception.

Colleges of optometry around the United States also established residency programs in the 1970s. The State University of New York's College of Optometry was the first to offer such a program, which consisted of a one year postgraduate didactic and clinical training in vision therapy. In the 1980s, several graduate-level programs in behavioral optometry were listed in the Residency Graduate Program Directory of the Association of Schools and Colleges of Optometry. The Southern California College of Optometry had a children's vision residency program; a master's of education degree in visual function in learning was created at Oregon's Pacific University College of Optometry; a pediatric optometry and vision therapy residency was at Southern College of Optometry in Memphis, Tennessee; and the E. B. Alexander Fellowship was founded at Connecticut's Gesell Institute.

The 1970s and 1980s saw the application of sophisticated technology to vision therapy. Optometry once again showed its ability to incorporate and adapt principles from other fields. The vision therapy of the second half of the twentieth century is the integration of many disciplines with the field of physiological optics. The therapy is spreading around the world, due to the dedication of American optometrists who travel ceaselessly and volunteer their time in nation after nation, including Australia, Belgium, China, France, Italy, Japan, Mexico, Spain, the Scandinavian countries and the nations of the Third World.

Vision & Behavior: The Unbreakable Link

In the early years when behavioral optometry was in its formative stages, optometric vision therapy was an innovative concept in its infancy. Not surprisingly, many of the papers on the history of optometric vision therapy in professional periodicals such as the *Journal of the American Optometric Association*, the *Journal of Optometric Vision Development* or the *Journal of Learning Disabilities* are in technical or professional language. The articles may read like lists of names and dates commemorating incomprehensible events. But because Dr. Skeffington involved so many leaders from other fields, some of the names are familiar to general readers. The name of Arnold Gesell, M.D., was virtually a household word for generations of parents, educators and counselors.

In a paper "Mileposts to Maturity" presented in 1971 in New Orleans to a meeting of the College of Optometrists in Vision Development, Dr. G. N. Getman, explains how it was that Dr. Gesell became involved in Dr. Skeffington's quest to establish that vision was a system that developed and could thus be trained. Widely regarded as one of the world's leading behaviorists and a specialist in child development, Dr. Gesell would eventually publish, with Drs. Ilg and Ames, a series of books on child development that would make the authors' names known in many countries. The Gesell Institute for Human Development had roots that went back to 1911 when Dr. Gesell founded his clinic for child study at Yale University.

In his paper, Dr. Getman explains how the research of educator Miss Glenna Bullis in the 1930s for an "examination and analysis to explain the magnitude of reading readiness she was observing in preschool children" led her to Dr. Bragden, a New Haven optometrist who eventually introduced Miss Bullis to Dr. Skeffington. At that time, Dr. Skeffington was searching "for a functional complex for the examination and analysis of near-point vision."

Shortly after this, Dr. Skeffington went to New Haven to meet Dr. Gesell. Over the next few years, at conferences and meetings, Dr. Skeffington and Dr. Gesell and their colleagues exchanged information from their various fields. It became clear that in the optometric approach being developed by the team led by Dr. Skeffington there was a total philosophy of vision which had importance for the Gesell philosophy of child development. Some of those prominent in optometry, Dr. George Crow and, in particular, members of the Missouri Valley Optometric Society like Dr. Ray Lowry, spent days and weeks at a time working with Dr. Gesell at Yale to help him understand the intricacies of the optometric philosophy being developed.

Then a situation arose that looked as though it would block progress. Under university rules, Dr. Gesell was due to retire. Finances, as ever, were also part of the picture. Enter optometrist Dr. Alexander. He went to work on the problem.

Dr. Getman wrote that Dr. Alexander and Walter Stewart, president of the American Optical Company in Massachusetts were good friends and Dr. Alexander took the problem to Mr. Stewart. After detailed conversations between Dr. Alexander, Dr. Skeffington and Mr. Stewart's board of directors, the sum of $100,000 was awarded by American Optical so that Dr. Gesell and his entire staff could stay on long enough to complete the studies of early visual development and write the book *Vision: Its Development in Infant and Child.* The early studies for this work had been funded by significant grants from various sources, including the Optometric Extension Program Foundation.

This book, published in 1949 by Harper & Brothers, was the result of an unusual collaboration. Dr. Gesell, was an internationally recognized authority on child behavior. Frances Ilg, M.D., was an ophthalmologist, Glenna Bullis, an educator, while G. N. Getman, Vivienne Ilg and George Crow were all distinguished optometrists. A seminal book, *Vision* paved the way for probing research into the connection between behavior and vision by the Gesell Institute's Department of Vision.

We See With Our Brains

The text of *Vision* explores the development of our vision systems from the time we are born. It offers a definition that stands intact decades later. Vision, explained Gesell et al., is a "complex sensory motor response to a light source mediated by the eyes but involving the whole action system."

Gesell and his team may have predated the work of Dr. Roger Sperry, the psychobiologist who shared the 1981 Nobel Prize for Medicine, but they were in perfect accord with him. Sperry, who has long advocated a holistic view of mind and body (a Gesell axiom), sees the brain as a mechanism for transforming sensory patterns into patterns of motor coordination. He argues that the major work of the visual system is to prepare the brain to respond to whatever the situation demands.

The following is adapted from *Vision.*

The Three Basic Areas of Your Body's Vision System

Skeletal: Your body's frame, the bones of your skeleton, are visually guided as well as directed. This means vision directs your body in:

Posture change	An example of this is when you
Searching	turn your body to watch a ball
Following	or someone running.

Visceral: Instinctive bodily reactions, guided by vision, help you concentrate your:

Attention	The visceral can be thought of as
Discrimination	a gut feeling which may be present
Definition	during problem solving.

Cortical: Your brain attempts, with the help of vision, to integrate all the available information simultaneously:

Identification	What is it?
Localization	Where is it?
Synthesis	Blending the information, so you can zero in.
Interpretation:	Your understanding of the information.

In his book, Gesell explained that:

The highest acts of vision are so interfused with cortical influences that they belong to the supreme realm of abstract thought.

Indeed, in the last analysis, the cortex becomes the seat of action for the action system. Sherrington [British Nobel-prize-winning neurophysiologist], Chavasse and Duke-Elders [M.D.s] all emphasize the fundamental role of body and limb movements in the mechanisms of vision.

Norman Cousins writes in his book, *Head First, the Biology of Hope:*

"Just in the past half-century...new findings have emphasized the glandular role of the brain. Indeed, new research suggests that the brain may be the most prolific gland in the human body. Some three dozen secretions are produced or activated by the brain. The brain also has the ability to combine these secretions, meaning that there are literally thousands of prescriptions the brain can write to meet the body's needs.... Endorphins and enkephalins may play a role in regulating immune function and tumor growth as well.

"The human brain serves as a control post for millions of messengers carrying instructions to the body's organs without intruding on the conscious intelligence. Recent research tends to emphasize 'communication' rather than 'connection' to describe the process by which the brain interacts with the body. This two-way communication system is as varied, complex, and busy as the operations of any air control tower at the world's largest airports."

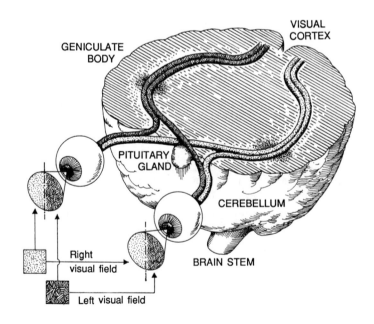

A simplified view of the vision system. The pathway from the eyes to the brain must be free of problems if one is to have accurate perceptions of what is happening.

By the 1970s, the Gesell Institute's Department of Vision was one of the bastions of optometry. It always had been. But in those early days, a major question faced Dr. Gesell and his staff. The team who had researched the subject of vision for the book included people who practiced optometry and ophthalmology. Each of those disciplines then and now offers routine eye care. It was clear to Gesell and his team that an additional dimension had been exposed. Which discipline was best suited to incorporate the care of the vision system into its practice?

One of the few people still at the Gesell Institute in 1985 from the years when the book *Vision* was being written was Louise B. Ames, Ph.D. A founding member, Dr. Ames had been one of the institute's associate directors for years. Dr. Ames, who is known around the world for her authorship and collaboration on a variety of books about child development, was still putting in long hours at the institute in 1985. But Dr. Ames made time for an interview with writer Hazel Richmond Dawkins to share the perspective of those early years.

In Whose Hands?

"When we first established the framework of the institute in 1948, we faced a difficult decision. The information in Doctor Gesell's book had brought us to a specific starting place. A major decision confronted us. Should we join the ophthalmologists or the optometrists?

"Arnold Gesell and Frances Ilg were both doctors of medicine. They were very serious in their consideration of joining ophthalmology. This was because ophthalmologists are doctors of medicine while optometrists are not. It was a great temptation to swing to the side of ophthalmology, but we finally clarified our position. Ophthalmology is essentially the detection of diseases or defects of the eye. We felt we could contribute to optometry.

"The final decision to join the side of optometry was nevertheless made with a certain amount of reluctance. In the 1940s, optometry did not have the respect of the medical profession.

Finally, however, our entire team resolved that it was important for us to work with doctors of optometry."

Dr. Ames recalled with a certain amount of amusement those early years. "Once the Gesell Institute was organized, Dr. Ilg and I began writing a syndicated newspaper column, 'Parents Ask.' This led to television and radio work. At one point in the early 1950s, we devoted some of the weekly columns to behavioral optometry and optometric vision therapy. Immediately, some members of the medical profession raised a terrible furor.

"The Gesell Institute received letters protesting the information in the column. Threats were made to revoke the institute's license. The fact was, of course, we didn't have a license because we didn't need one.

"After that, whenever I mentioned behavioral optometry in a lecture, caustic reactions from the audience invariably came from medical practitioners."

World War II--Vision Is Needed

Dr. Getman wrote that World War II was "a war where there was a new recognition of visual ability as contrasted to visual acuity [clarity of sight]. Many optometrists were discovering visual training because of the demand from young men to pass the acuity charts of the various services. The optometrists who had explored and accepted the functional philosophy being taught by Dr. Skeffington found they could do something for these young men.... Visual training became a part of many optometric practices, and the accumulated records show that several thousand men went into service after previous rejection because of low acuity."

By the 1980s, that aspect of optometric vision therapy, the reduction of nearsightedness, was well established. Whether for the national program for space exploration, military endeavors or careers in aviation or law enforcement, men and women who had failed entrance exams because of symptoms such as nearsightedness found that through optometric vision therapy they were able to change and improve their vision, retake exams and pass.

Dr. Skeffington and his colleagues might not have foreseen the total range and scope of the therapy they were meticulously developing. Could they have known that their pioneering work would lead to help for an astoundingly diverse range of situations? In those early years, they were certain that those whose vision imbalances triggered headaches or backaches or difficulties with learning or behavior would be helped by the procedures they were developing. Did they suspect that optometric vision therapy would help juvenile delinquents, dyslexics, schizophrenics or cerebral palsy victims? All that is certain is that the scientific studies then and now have corroborated their work.

160,000 School-children In Texas

Two questions are usually asked about optometric vision therapy when a youngster is having difficulty in school but has 20/20 sight. Why and how do you know such a therapy is necessary? The early research concentrated on this type of proof. A study was made in the early 1940s by the Texas Department of Public Health. It involved 160,000 schoolchildren in 4,000 classrooms. The study showed that some 20 percent of the youngsters entering school had clinically measurable vision imbalances. This figure increased to 40 percent some two and a half years later. At the end of fifth grade, as many as 80 percent of the students had developed vision imbalances.

Stress & the Avoidance Response

As the researchers interpreted the results of this study, they were able to identify the various reasons for the jump in numbers. One was what behavioral optometry believes to be one of the most significant reactions we have to stress; it is defined as the avoidance response. A study by Dr. Harmon at the Radiological Group laboratory in Austin, Texas, yielded important filmed evidence of the avoidance response while reading. In 1950, the film made of this for educators was widely regarded as being of prime importance.

Youngsters and adults who are reading material that's difficult for them have back tension; their heads and necks oscillate; blood pressure fluctuates; respiration increases and the galvanic skin response is abnormal. As the technology in the field improved, electrophysiological studies reproduced and validated Dr. Harmon's first study.

These body tensions are incredibly stressful reactions to endure. In turn, the effect of such stress on the vision system is considerable. Dr. V. Shipman wrote in one of the Optometric Extension Program Foundation's pamphlets for parents and teachers that under the stress caused by the avoidance response, peripheral vision is reduced, literally constricted. This "leads to perceptual loss and the child or adult observes less, sees less, remembers less, and becomes generally less efficient."

In a June 1970 article in the *Journal of Vision Development*, Dr. L. Stevens of California wrote that "nervous strain produces stress that changes structure. Tension movements are opposed by the same amount of antagonistic...contraction. It's like driving your car with the brakes partly on."

Stress & Biochemical & Biophysical Changes

Once research had proved that difficult work leads to hormonal and biophysical alterations, the next step was to establish how behavioral optometry could help. At this point, the way behavioral optometrists use lenses and prisms showed its value. A certain type of lens, which does not seem very powerful when the lay person or the uninitiated examines it, can literally relieve the stress produced by reading difficult material or trying to learn to read.

Stress-Reducing Lenses:

Lenses used in optometric vision therapy to help lessen stress are called convex, spherical plus lenses. Electrophysiological studies have shown that when such a lens is worn, the results are dramatic. Even though the individual was working hard visually, back tensions reduced, neck and head oscillations stopped, blood pressure, respiration and galvanic skin response returned to normal.

In chapters 5 and 6, you can read about the ways in which lens use in optometric vision therapy is drastically different from lens use by general optometrists and ophthalmologists. This variance evolved because the philosophies and perspectives of behavioral optometry and ophthalmology are at different ends of the spectrum, with one (the optometric specialty) treating the causes of vision imbalances and the other (ophthalmology) believing that such treatment is not possible and in general working with symptoms only. The essential factor is that optometric vision therapy is preventive health care.

The next section, Illogical Barriers, explains why so many people have not heard about this therapy, even though it has been offered as a health therapy for decades. Few books have been written about optometric vision therapy for the general reader (see the list in Recommended Reading). The American Optometric Association, the College of Optometrists in Vision Development and the Optometric Extension Program Foundation publish valuable pamphlets, but these are mostly distributed by optometrists to their patients. The general public is rarely aware that such material exists. Coupled with this is a virtual lack of consumer education. The professional organizations focus on professional education, a reasonable approach since their funds are limited.

One of the main obstacles to public awareness has been the opposition of traditional medicine, which claims, wrongly, that this optometric therapy lacks scientific research and documentation. The research does exist and is both scientific and documented. Fortunately, the people who have benefited are uniformly enthusiastic and supportive; indeed, most referrals are from patients who have benefited from the therapy. Another telling point is that health insurance does cover it. Yet considerable resistance still exists and from a group which has one of the most powerful and well-funded lobbies in the country, the American Medical Association. New York optometrist Dr. Richard S. Kavner, author of two of the best books on optometric vision therapy for the general reader, *Total Vision* and *Your Child's Vision*, has noted that traditional medicine shows a reluctance even to debate the issue.

Illogical Barriers

"I know that most men--not only those considered clever, but even those who are clever and capable of understanding the most difficult scientific, mathematical, or philosophic problems--can seldom discern even the simplest and most obvious truth if it be such as obliges them to admit the falsity of conclusions they have formed, perhaps with much difficulty--conclusions of which they are proud, which they have taught to others, and on which they have built their lives." Leo Tolstoy, 1898.

This perceptive paragraph is as true now as when Tolstoy first wrote it. But in fact, scientific "gospel" is being redefined today. "There was a time when doctors scoffed at the idea that certain enigmatic diseases might be caused by bacteria," wrote L. K. Altman, M.D., in the *New York Times* of February 14, 1984. "After all, they reasoned, the laboratory methods of detecting bacteria had been so standard for so long [1850, when medical microscopy developed] that it seemed unlikely any organisms could have been missed. But to their surprise in recent years, doctors have learned that bacteria cause legionnaire's disease and Lyme arthritis, and they are now proposing to add cat scratch disease to the list of bacterial infections."

Our horizons must continually expand for new concepts. Yet there is always the resistance of the old establishment. In art they resisted Picasso. In music they resisted Wagner. In science, Pasteur. Einstein's theories produced storms of fury in the world community of scientists. Many hadn't the flexibility to consider his unconventional work.

In the mid-1880s, Ignatz Semmelweiss, M.D., believed that childbed fever, widespread and deadly, could be ended by a simple precaution. "Wash your hands before you assist at childbirth," he implored his fellow practitioners. Their reaction was inflexible. "Waste of time," they retorted.

Waste of money, too, they thought, even though Semmelweiss arranged for buckets of soapy water to be placed at the foot of beds in the maternity ward. Up to that time, Semmelweiss had been an influential gynecologist-obstetrician. He was a prominent member of society and a distinguished member of the medical establishment. For years he preached his case against germs--and it ruined him.

Semmelweiss became an outcast and, eventually, a suicide. Time and history vindicated him. The story of Semmelweiss is not unique. The physician who devised the stethoscope was ridiculed and humiliated and his invention ignored for decades. What physician today would go without a stethoscope? It is notoriously the fate of the innovator to be ignored or condemned. The prophet-without-honor syndrome operates in all ages.

This Therapy is Another Health Tool

Today's optometrists who practice optometric vision therapy face the same resistance to innovation, although their therapy adds another tool to our health care resources. Despite all efforts, countries like the United States have many with chronic health problems, although they have sought help from a range of practitioners. We also have many who have difficulty fitting their behavior into the framework we define as "normal." In schools, the remedial education and special classes have not been as successful as hoped; far too many students have difficulty learning to read in the early grades and, by the time they leave school, are still not reading adequately.

In *Illiterate America,* author Jonathan Kozol cites appalling figures. Sixty million adults, a third of America's population, cannot read a daily newspaper, while 22 percent of adults cannot write a check or address an envelope. Illiteracy costs the US government and taxpayers about $120 billion annually, with an additional $100 billion in lowered GNP. Also, 60 percent of prison inmates and 85 percent of juvenile delinquents are unable to read.

Numerous research projects have established that optometric vision therapy is a valuable remedy for illiteracy, for it has succeeded where other therapies have failed.

Rebuttal Based on Fact

When examined carefully, the resistance to optometric vision therapy is as much the traditional distrust of something new and different as it is an economic situation. Perhaps another factor is that ophthalmology considers the therapy overlaps territory to which they claim possession: eye care. In 1984, a panel of behavioral optometrists, Drs. Nathan Flax, Rochelle Mozlin and Harold Solan, wrote an editorial in the *Journal of the American Optometric Association* which documented errors in a position paper published by an ad hoc working group of the American Association for Pediatric Ophthalmology and the American Academy of Ophthalmology (Appendixes II and III).

A complaint by ophthalmology is that little research exists to verify optometric vision therapy. Apparently, the scrutiny of the researchers for the ophthalmologic paper did not include the professional journals of optometry. Of course, not all ophthalmologists support the stand by their academy, which first issued a policy statement denying any relationship between vision and learning in 1972. There are ophthalmologists who know of and value optometric vision therapy.

Pediatricians, too, are sometimes disinclined to refer patients for optometric vision therapy because in general they follow the lead of the ophthalmologists, their peers in medicine. Again, fortunately, there are pediatricians who have seen firsthand the valuable results of the therapy and who do not hesitate to endorse it for their patients. The impact of the general resistance is still considerable, however. What actually are the differences between ophthalmology and behavioral optometry?

Different Perspectives

Many of the terms and descriptions used in optometry are the same as those used in ophthalmology. The critical difference lies in the interpretation of the situation and the treatment. Optometrists who practice optometric vision therapy believe that vision imbalances, including nearsightedness, astigmatism, eyes that cross or turn out or up, or nystagmoid oscillation can be helped because they are adaptations that the individual has made. Such adaptations usually can be reversed or modified. Further, behavioral optometrists believe that the individual adapts, causes changes in physical structure and uses various strategies in order to meet demands or needs. Under stress, which may be self-induced, the individual makes maladaptations--nearsightedness, or eyes that cross, or a lazy eye. People will sacrifice efficient ways for less efficient ones to create an easier way of functioning.

Here it's important to realize that the decision to adapt or change ways of functioning takes place at a subconscious level. You can compare this to increased blood pressure. Perhaps it is your body's reaction to stress or diet. Whatever the trigger, your body reacts in a specific way. It is this type of biological adaptation which the behavioral optometrist is describing. On the other hand, ophthalmology for the most part believes you must live with most of your vision problems because heredity, genetics, your luck-in-the-draw have determined and created a rigid framework. Under the rules of ophthalmology, you can expect to wear heavier and heavier lenses if you are nearsighted, although in the late 1980s, surgery was promoted for some nearsighted individuals. The option of optometric vision therapy for nearsightedness is not widely known.

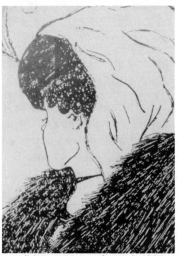

It is possible to see two faces in this art, although you cannot see both at the same time. One is an attractive woman in profile, while the other woman is in three-quarter profile and has a large, hooked nose and a thin, curved chin.

In the above illustration you see the two faces alternately, which is how the brain achieves visual concentration. Visual information is organized by excluding competing information. Individuals who have difficulty with this type of distrimination are likely to have trouble concentrating on written information. This picture, known as "Wife-Mistress," was devised by a psychologist.

Working With Nystagmoid Oscillation

If you had nystagmoid oscillation, you might well be given contrasting diagnoses by optometry and ophthalmology. An oscillation or involuntary movement brought on by drugs or alcohol cannot be controlled voluntarily, which is why police in the United States use the nystagmus gaze test to check drivers whose actions seem suspicious. But if your vision system develops a nystagmoid oscillation as a result of macula degeneration or optic atrophy, optometric vision therapy can often help. Such an oscillation may be large or small, it may go up, down, round or sideways. The cause of it may be organic, that is, damage to the neurological system may have caused it. Or the cause may be functional, because the individual is trying to find the light and has learned (subconsciously) to move the eye quickly, or oscillate it.

An oscillation occurs when the vision system loses control of a regular pattern and the eye movement fluctuates from the smooth normal movement. Some oscillations can be seen just by looking at the individual, others cannot be seen with the naked eye and must be detected by special tests.

Optometric vision therapy is unique in that it has had good results treating the nystagmoid oscillation in individuals of all ages. Young patients treated for nystagmus frequently had behavior and learning problems which had been triggered by the oscillation; adults had similar problems and a high level of tension and anxiety. When the therapy helped these individuals gain a better balance in their vision systems and reduce or eliminate the oscillation, their other problems were responsive to other therapies or education and also improved or disappeared.

A nystagmoid oscillation can be reduced when the individual gains an internal control of the visual skills such as eye movement and teaming. Some describe this as biofeedback. Optometric vision therapy is designed to help the individual develop control of the way their vision system works.

"Our daughter doesn't look at us."

When Jan and Ed Baker had their second child, they were delighted to have a daughter. Their firstborn, John, was a robust four-year-old, happy to welcome his sister home. It took a few weeks but the Bakers noticed that Susan never made eye contact with them, yet their son had and they had seen that other infants did. They also noticed that their baby's eyes jerked back and forth. Visits to several specialists, including those at one of America's leading eye institutions, brought the news that Susan's jerky eye movement was a severe case of nystagmus. Nothing was recommended to help improve the child's poor vision.

The Bakers lived with their concern until they were eventually referred to optometrist Dr. Getman, whose associate Dr. Beth Ballinger handled the case. When Susan was first seen by Dr. Ballinger at her office in Newport Beach, California, she was a hesitant, nervous child. She did not run and play like other youngsters her age. The parents told Dr. Ballinger that if Susan was going from the kitchen to the living room, which involved walking from tile to carpet, the little girl would hesitate and slide her feet across the floor to check if the level was different. Her vision was so poor she could not see that the floor was flat. She could tell that the surface had changed only because of the color difference.

The Bakers were astonished but delighted when Dr. Ballinger said that she could develop a program to help Susan. In addition to monthly office visits, Susan's parents worked at home daily using procedures prescribed by the optometrist. Some three months after optometric vision therapy started, the change in Susan's vision and behavior was impressive. Gone was the nervous, hesitant child who did not run or play with her toys. Susan no longer shuffled around the house but ran confidently from room to room. She enjoyed playing with her toys and looks directly at her family.

"When we used to ask her if she could see the dog out in the backyard, we never got an answer. We'd been told she probably never would see beyond a few feet. Now, she tells us all about the birds and trees that she sees in the backyard as well as the dog," her mother said. "It's hard to believe it's the same child. We had a daughter who was so slow and nervous. Not any more. Now, she's as outgoing and confident as her brother."

Susan's nystagmus was soon brought under control and eventually it reached the point where it did not interfere with the function of the vision system.

No drugs, no surgery.

Fifteen Years of Physical Pain and Learning Difficulty

Anne Hamilton was not as fortunate as little Susan. She did not have optometric vision therapy recommended until she was twenty-six and had had four operations on her eyes.

Dr. Leonard Press, the optometrist who treated her, explained that her left eye had nystagmus and did not move smoothly with the right eye. Anne learned, in therapy with Dr. Press, to control the nystagmus to the point where it did not interfere with her processing of visual information.

Before therapy the effort she'd had to make to focus so she could see clearly had caused major physical pain and tension; it had also caused Anne's eyes to turn in. She frequently had double or blurred vision and her eyes were often bloodshot. Generally, she felt enormously tired.

Ophthalmology had tried both orthoptics and prism glasses but Anne still had all the same symptoms. In fact, everything seemed worse when she wore the glasses prescribed; this was because they were not correct for her needs. Eventually, surgery was recommended. Anne had four operations, all of which left her in a progressively worse state visually, physically and emotionally.

"Before each operation, I would be excited and hopeful that this time would be different, that I would be helped. After, I'd be depressed because I would feel even more uncomfortable. I still couldn't see properly, I still felt pain and tension, and I still hadn't been helped. Yet the doctors and my family told me I had been helped."

The constant tensing and focusing of her vision system in an effort to see clearly grew worse after each of the four operations. By the time she was twenty-six, Anne had endured years of pain and the emotional pressure of "experts" telling her to "live with it" because they had done all that was necessary. She felt at odds with her family, because they believed they had offered her the best possible health care. Perhaps much of the trouble was psychological, they suggested. And because she was always struggling to stay in school and could never play sports, Anne felt isolated from her peers and left out.

When a friend who'd benefited greatly from optometric vision therapy wrote and shared the news, Anne decided she had to explore this new avenue, even though her family cautioned her against doing so and suggested that the problem was in her mind, since surgery had been pronounced successful. Anne made her choice. Shortly after starting therapy at the Pennsylvania College of Optometry with Dr. Press (who moved to the State University of New York College of Optometry in the 1980s), Anne was able to learn to move her left eye more smoothly. Gradually, as she brought the nystagmoid oscillation under control, the symptoms of pain and tension subsided and her emotional distress lessened. Today, whenever she feels discomfort in her eyes (usually, stress is the trigger), she practices the procedures that have brought relief in the past.

Ultimately, counseling also was of value to Anne. She is no longer upset over her family's attitude. Rather, she can understand that their perspective is different from hers and that she had every right to seek therapy that would bring her some relief.

A Career Turnaround After Therapy

Mark Robertson is now thirty-four. His ophthalmologist in New York had diagnosed a nystagmoid oscillation when Mark was in grade school, which is also when Mark started wearing contact lenses. Chronically nearsighted, Mark had had "difficulty" with his eyes all his life. His right eye "wandered out" now and then; his eyes were often red and tired; he tilted his head when trying to read a book and could not see objects or faces in the distance. His general coordination was poor and he was bothered by normal amounts of light.

When Mark started optometric vision therapy with Dr. Edelman, as a first step, the optometrist cut the prescription for nearsightedness in half. Therapy was begun to help Mark learn to control the oscillation in his right eye. Mark also listed his goals. He wanted to:

- drive a car comfortably

- not be anxious when entering a new environment

- see a person's face before someone reached him

- recognize people by their faces

- be able to make eye contact

- increase physical confidence

When Mark started wearing his new prescription contact lenses, Dr. Edelman told him to expect rapid changes in his physical tension. Mark noticed a difference by the second day but a few days later, he was astounded to realize the level of change.

"By the fifth day of wearing my new contacts, my usual anxiety and tension was cut in half. I had never realized just how much tension I was under from my vision problems," Mark says. "But the really incredible change took place with my career. After I began treatment with Dr. Edelman, I started up another contracting business, even though the first had failed.

"I'd been in the vision therapy and wearing the milder lenses for about eight months when I began the second effort. In my first year of operation, my income was in the six figures and the business grossed $3 million. My wife and I know that there's no way I could have handled the pressure of creating and running the business before the therapy."

Mark and his wife also explain that he gained personal confidence and stability with the lessening of his vision imbalance.

"My friends used to joke that I lived on short notice," says Mark. "They were right, that was how I managed. I just could not see far ahead. Now, I look at the concepts, at the overall picture. My anxiety level has gone down dramatically. I have a different awareness when I am on the road in my car. I'm more aware of a wider range when driving. I've reached my goals and more, because I see differently and think differently and perceive differently."

Mark first heard about optometric vision therapy through a friend in New York, whose music teacher had been so severely visually handicapped that she had had to learn to use Braille. Until she was taken to Dr. Richard Kavner, the woman had virtually existed as a blind person. Optometric vision therapy changed that. Mark's wife, a teacher, had several students at her school show dramatic changes after therapy with Dr. Edelman.

"When my wife came home and suggested I visit Dr. Edelman to find out if the therapy the children had received would work for me I remembered the incredible changes that happened to the supposedly blind music teacher in New York. What did I have to lose by trying it?" Mark said. "The results were spectacular, far beyond our hopes."

Not A Magic Answer

No one therapy is the answer for every ailment. Optometric vision therapy cannot help everyone. Each person's problems are unique. But when a vision imbalance is triggering problems, and where the individual has motivation, this is a therapy that can bring about substantial changes and improvements at many levels.

Good Sight, Terrible Vision

"Doctor, this is Mary Evans I'm telephoning to ask you to come speak to our PTA group. I'm the principal of the school that Andy Day attends. We're a small private school just outside Philadelphia, not far from your office at Newtown Square. Andy's parents tell me that the boy is your patient. Here at school we've all noticed such a change in Andy since you started treating him. We're hoping you will be able to explain to us how you helped Andy."

"I'm happy to accept your invitation," Dr. Edelman replied. "And I'm very glad to hear of Andy's improvements."

The principal laughed. "He gave new meaning to the word hyperactive. But now he's a different boy. Just what is it that you do?"

"I gave Andy the tools he needed, and he's using them."

"Yes, the parents explained the glasses he's wearing are most important. But we're puzzled because until now, his regular eye checks showed 20/20 sight."

"Oh, yes," Dr. Edelman agreed. "Andy's sight is fine. It's his vision that needs help. The glasses I prescribed for him are designed to reduce the stress on his vision system and to help the system develop in a balanced way. I treat the entire vision system, not just eye sight. My practice is devoted to optometric vision therapy. This work is broadly labeled behavioral because the way your vision system functions affects your behavior."

"Andy certainly had a behavior problem and it did affect his ability to learn," the principal said thoughtfully. "This is all amazing. I hope you will have a free evening soon to come and share news of this exciting work with our school."

"Of course," Dr. Edelman agreed.

In this brief conversation, Dr. Edelman had shared two key facts with the school principal.

1. Sight and vision are different.

2. Optometric vision therapy treats the entire vision system and the results affect learning and behavior.

"I feel so stupid. I've been staring at that slide for two minutes and I still don't know what it is."

The speaker is the principal who'd invited Dr. Edelman to talk about his work with the student Andy. A few of the faculty and parents at the crowded meeting murmur agreement. Others laugh nervously. Everyone seems to be completely puzzled by the slide Dr. Edelman is showing them.

Dr. Edelman had invited me, as the writer of this book, to join him at the school for the evening's talk. Amazed at the comments, I look at the large screen. When the slide had been displayed, ten times larger than I'd ever seen it, I'd groaned mentally. Who could fail to recognize the slide immediately? Surely the whole point of using this picture would be ruined now. The animal shown on the slide was so clear to me, how could anyone else, particularly a group of savvy teachers, fail to identify the slide? The audience sat in puzzled silence when Dr. Edelman asked what animal was pictured on the slide.

When the principal confessed she was baffled, Dr. Edelman's reply completed my surprise. He did not identify the picture but commented on an issue that meant a lot to everyone there that evening.

"Now you know how some of your students feel. They can see the work you give them quite clearly, but they don't know what it is. They feel stupid, too. Sometimes they are told the work isn't hard and they should be able to do it. This doesn't help their confidence or self-image."

When Dr. Edelman had suggested I join him at the school meeting, I'd agreed cheerfully. Our paperback, *The Suddenly Successful Student, A Guide to Overcoming Learning & Behavior Problems* had just come out. Dr. Edelman asked if I would talk about the book when his lecture finished. As its writer, I had started to promote the paperback with radio and television interviews and talks to groups. I was in the fortunate position of being able to discuss the therapy from various viewpoints: a patient who'd had the therapy, a writer who had exhaustively researched the subject, and a wife and parent whose husband and four of the family's five children had benefited from the therapy.

When we used the slide in postcard form at health fairs and conferences like the one I'd recently attended for dyslexia, few people could identify the picture, even after looking at it for several minutes. Occasionally, artists would put a name on it, but it would take even their trained eyes a while. Some people even had difficulty recognizing the picture after they'd been told what the card showed. This was exactly what was happening at the school meeting described above. Quite a few people called out that they still didn't see what the picture was, even when Dr. Edelman identified it. Test yourself. Can you recognize what the following picture shows?

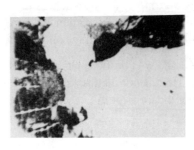

Figure 1. Can You Identify This?

This is a picture of a well-known object. It may not be clear to you what it is, but think of this: you can see the picture clearly, although you may lack understanding of what it is.

Several factors are involved when you look at Figure 1 (or anything). You have to know, visually, where something is, and you have to scan. You know you are looking at the picture if your eyes are pointing at it. Then, after we know where, we scan for familiar shapes. We can agree that the picture has masses of gray and no sharp edges.

As Dr. Edelman explained at that school meeting, the reason few people identify the picture easily is that although you see the picture clearly, until your vision system integrates the whole, you do not understand the picture. Now look at the next picture on the following page.

This picture has lines added to it which may help you identify what it shows. If you're having difficulty identifying it, you'll find the answer in the following paragraph.

Did the lines drawn on the second picture help you realize that this is the picture of a cow? Once you recognize it, if you look back at the first picture, which was so puzzling, it's clear it's a cow. Some people object that this is a visual puzzle. Life isn't like that, they say. But it's true that sometimes when we first look at something, we fail to identify it until we've put all the clues into place through our vision system. The cow "test" was devised by Dr. Samuel Renshaw, an experimental psychologist who worked

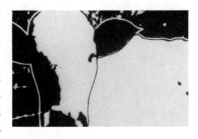

Figure 2. Do the Lines Help?

closely with the pioneers of optometric vision therapy. It isn't presented as a trick. It's a simple but effective demonstration of one of the core concepts of optometric vision therapy: sight and vision are different.

At first, although you could see Figure 1 clearly, you probably did not know what it was. Once your entire vision system has made the identification, it will be able to retrieve the information each time you look at the picture. That's vision, the ability to guide us through our world, to integrate what we see into meaningful information. Your acuity or clarity did not change from the first time you looked at the picture until it was explained to you what it was. But your comprehension of the information did.

Many practitioners of optometric vision therapy use the Renshaw cow picture to help people understand what is meant by vision. Coauthor Dr. Forkiotis often includes it in his talks to officer candidates for the Connecticut State Police.

Police officers are trained to evaluate at speed. Sometimes their lives or the lives of others depend on how quickly the police can react. A balanced vision system brings accuracy to the police officer's speedy reaction.

Chapter 3

Everyone Needs Vision Skills --Not Everyone Has Them

Our vision systems are akin to a blank sheet of paper when we are infants. We must learn to use our eyes and our vision systems so that we can have eye-brain-behavior communication. All our early life centers on our learning to connect sight with understanding. Many different visual skills are involved. Clear sight is not enough. Understanding is the key and vision plays the major role in understanding. The development of the vision system from infancy to adulthood is an ongoing process. Parents and educators can help to make sure that each step of this development has as much support as possible. If visual skills are not learned in childhood, then the adult will lack them, too. Remember, while your eyesight may be wonderful, your vision can be terrible.

When the vision system is balanced, you can:

1. Use both eyes together as a team (binocular ability)

2. Focus the eyes quickly and accurately (accommodative ability)

3. Know where objects are in space (spatial judgment)

4. React with accurate mind-body response to actions 1 through 3 above; that is, have the ability to solve problems and move through space accurately

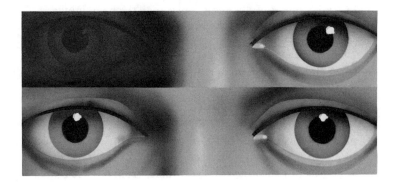

This art represents one of the most important abilities of the vision system: teaming. If your teaming is inadequate, your perception of what is going on around you is not accurate.

A significant proportion of us lack one or more of these abilities. Yet without them, it is impossible to lead a normal productive life without enormous extra stress being placed on your body. You cannot function up to your potential. You're leaking energy through your eyes!

We have a team of interacting visual skills as well as the four basic visual abilities listed above. All can be learned as part of the growing-up process. Often they are not. They include:

1. *Clearness of vision (acuity)* The ability to see clearly at near and far distances. (Clarity at distance is usually the only skill tested by the conventional eyechart exam.) If you score 20/20 on a Snellen eyechart that means you see clearly for distance sight; your near distance clarity needs to be tested separately.

   Generally, people who have poor distance acuity are nearsighted; they can handle reading but fare less well at sports.

   The farsighted person tends to have more difficulty reading, but often does better at sports than the nearsighted.

2. *Dynamic visual acuity* The ability to see sharply and clearly while an object or person is in motion. This is vital to an athlete but we are all athletes to some degree. When we drive or walk across a street or use an escalator, we must clearly see other cars, other people in motion, the curbs, handrails and starting and stopping places. Without visual pursuit skills, you can't follow a ball in flight. You can't move your eyes smoothly across a line of text on a page. A child can't shift the eyes accurately from a close object to a far one, such as from a notebook to a blackboard.

3. *Peripheral vision* The ability to use side vision. Without it, you can't be a quarterback and you shouldn't be driving a car.

4. *Eye-movement skills* The ability to make swift and accurate eye movements from one object to another.

5. *Eye-teaming skills* Converging and diverging. The ability to turn the eyes inward or outward, looking from objects close up to objects far away and back again. These skills must be closely coordinated with eye-focusing skills and eye movement. Inadequacies seriously hamper reading ability and athletic performance.

6. *Binocular fusion* The ability to coordinate and align the eyes precisely so that the brain can fuse the input. Even a slight imbalance here will cause trouble.

In some cases, when the eyes don't team, you get double vision which in turn may lead to the brain suppressing the use of one eye. The brain reacts in a disturbed and defensive manner to confusing signals from the eyes.

7. *Eye-hand coordination* The ability of the vision system (eye-brain communication) to coordinate the information received through the eyes in order to monitor and direct the hands.

8. *Visual form perception* The ability to organize images on the printed page into letters and/or words. It is one of the most important skills used in learning to read and is developed through both experience and practice.

9. *Eye-focusing skills* The ability to make rapid and accurate shifts in visual inspection with instantaneous clarity at any distance. It also relates to the ease or efficiency with which visual attention can be sustained.

All these skills can be taught, developed or improved.

An Olympic Champion

You don't have to have learning or behavior problems to benefit from optometric vision therapy, although it came as news to US Olympian Anita Miller of Pennsylvania that she could learn to see better. Off the experience of a lifetime of athletics, she thought she saw very well indeed. Bright, bouncy, scattering smiles on all sides as she goes her way, Anita moves like the athlete she is. You expect her to have good eyesight. Anita is a triple threat.

She has a master's degree in Administration of Physical Education, holds the position of Athletic Director of Bryn Mawr's Academy of the Sacred Heart where she coaches hockey; during the summer hiatus she is the Director and Head Coach of the Field Hockey Camp at Sacred Heart Academy. She has a national reputation as an equestrian. She is also a world-class field hockey player, a member of the US Olympic Field Hockey team that brought home a bronze medal from the

1984 games. A 1982-83 Co-Athlete of the Year in Field Hockey, Anita has been inducted into the Hall of Fame at Ohio University.

Anita does have both superior eyesight and superior vision. Nevertheless, she and other members of her Olympic team took extensive optometric vision therapy as part of their preparations for the Olympic Games. This is the kind of training that makes good athletes better.

Fundamentally, Anita was surprised to learn of the difference between sight and vision. She had assumed that her 20/20 performance on the eye charts meant that her vision had no room for improvement. Then she discovered optometric vision therapy. Twice a week for some six months, Miller and her teammates took part in a sports vision program.

"I was interested in how useful vision care proved to my daily life," says Anita. "It helped my driving, my peripheral vision, my perception of events. I still use some of the procedures we learned, just to keep up the level of my vision. When we were away or on tour, we all used to practice what we had learned in the vision training."

It is noteworthy that Anita Miller had the most consistently superior vision skills of all the athletes tested up to 1984 at the center where she took the optometric vision therapy. When she had a routine vision analysis in 1985 by Dr. Edelman, he found that she had the most balanced vision system he had ever examined.

Here is the vision skills profile for Anita:

Eye tracking	Very good
Accommodation	Above average
(Less flexible than desirable for her needs)	
Binocular fusion (eye teaming)	Very good +
Stereopsis (depth perception)	Excellent
Peripheral awareness	Very good +
Visual reaction time	Very good +
Eye-hand coordination	Very good ++

| Visualization | Very good +++ |
| Spatial localization | Very good ++++ |

Accommodation, the ability of the eyes to change focus quickly and accurately, was Anita's weak point--although calling her accommodation weak is like complaining when Superwoman takes two seconds instead of one to leap mighty buildings in a bound. Optometric vision therapy brought strength to Anita's accommodation. It actually brought improvement to her strong points.

Like Anita Miller, many American athletes, amateur and professional, have come to depend on sports vision care to give them their extra edge in competition. Optometric vision therapy is valuable when it comes to honing good skills to a fine edge. Tuning up the visual system pays dividends even when it's a superior system. But what happens to the average system when it is time to go to kindergarten?

A Suddenly Successful Student

Joanna's story is classic. The trouble she found herself in because of her vision difficulty is not uncommon. Joanna's chronological age and her vision developmental age were out of step. This presented a problem that would get worse as time went on. Five years old, in kindergarten, Joanna was emotionally mature, liked by her classmates and socially well-adjusted. Yet her teacher, a veteran of many past kindergarten classes, discovered there was something going seriously wrong with Joanna.

Despite the child's best efforts to learn to read, and despite her ready intelligence, she was getting nowhere. The teacher discovered that Joanna couldn't tell the difference between B, D and P. The youngster was becoming frustrated by her lack of success and by the progress the others made while she floundered.

When the report card went home at the end of the first term, the teacher wrote: "I fear Joanna may develop a lack of confidence as well as fall behind."

The irony in this situation is that Joanna is the granddaughter of a behavioral optometrist. Her grandfather had checked Joanna's vision system regularly since birth. Joanna's mother had actually worked for several years as an assistant in a behavioral optometrist's office. Joanna had had routine checks as she grew--and one before starting school, something recommended for every child. Until she started kindergarten, all had been developing well but then the situation changed. The pressure of trying to learn to read with a vision system which was not adequately developed for such a task caused stress to the vision system. This stress forms a barrier to learning.

When Joanna's parents read the report card, they immediately took their daughter to the grandfather for a vision analysis. As a first step, the developmental level of the child's vision system was measured. And the answer to Joanna's struggles leaped out. Despite her chronological age of 5 years, 4 months, Joanna's vision system was similar to that of a 4 year, 9 month old. The child was just not quite ready to read; trying to learn was a strain on her vision system.

Joanna's eyes had not finished learning to t*eam* or work together. This meant her vision system could not organize or put into any useful sequence what she tried to read. She might perceive THE as EHT. Sometimes it even seemed that the letters were upside down. These were the perceptions of her vision system. Astigmatism (the unequal curvature of the cornea) had developed in one eye as a result of her intense efforts to learn. She was developing an overconvergence (a tendency for the eyes to turn in because the vision system was pulling in when she tried to focus on reading at an early age). As a result, she held reading matter too close.

All this sounds serious. It had the potential to be and it had certainly given Joanna some unhappy months in kindergarten. The answer was clear. Joanna's grandfather prescribed glasses for nearpoint work such as reading. The lenses in the glasses were of a special kind, known as *developmental*. Whereas the conventional eye doctor prescribes *compensating* lenses that force the eyes to focus, the behavioral optometrist prescribes *developmental* lenses designed to relieve visual stress and help the whole vision system develop in a balanced way. *Compensating* lenses do not generally treat the causes of eye problems the way *developmental* lenses do. In fact, the compensating lens matches the visual distortion, such as nearsightedness or astigmatism. It does not help to change the individual's skew but merely compensates for the distortion. This ultimately perpetuates the problem.

Now that Joanna's vision system had help, there were dramatic changes at school. She was able to follow instructions and soon began to learn to read. The youngster was thrilled by her own progress and gradually grew confident of her ability. Her teacher said that she had only once before seen so dramatic a change in a youngster's learning ability. It was in a child who had also been to Joanna's grandfather and had been given developmental lenses to wear just for close work. Today, Joanna is a self-assured, cheerful schoolgirl, comfortable in her classes.

What Were the Benefits For Joanna?

What might have happened if this youngster had not received the necessary help for her vision imbalance? It almost certainly could have taken her far longer than the average to learn to read and, consequently, to learn. As a result of her struggle, Joanna would undoubtedly have developed a poor self image, low confidence and nagging frustrations. She probably would also have missed some schoolwork and not developed good powers of concentration or organizational skills. Her vision system would also have been affected by the stress of the situation. Because she would have been struggling to keep up with her peers, she would have continued to develop astigmatism. Nearsightedness might also have developed as her vision system sought to accommodate to its imbalance. Difficulties with her various vision skills could well develop and make it harder and harder for her to cope with school and family.

Altogether, not a very happy picture. It would get worse because the longer youngsters have to struggle with vision imbalances, the further behind they are likely to fall in school. They will need remedial education for what they've missed and, often, some kind of counselling to help them get over the feelings of inadequacy and frustration they have developed. If their vision dysfunctions are not treated, the remedial education and counselling will be of minimal value, perhaps even increase the tension and frustration. Stress on the vision system usually leads to further distortions that compound the original problems.

How Many Joannas?

Are vision imbalances common to school-age children or are they relatively rare? The American Optometric Association says that nearly 1 in 5 of the elementary school-children in the United States have vision imbalances that can hamper their learning and development.

Inadequate School Testing

The traditional eye testing done in most schools is usually based on the Snellen eye chart, which dates back to the 1860s. Sometimes a few other basic tests are also used. Regretfully, these tests only touch on a fraction of the skills that are needed for our vision systems to handle academic work adequately. A study in Texas in 1973 found that only 48 percent of the state's private schools screened their pupils' vision and more than half of those relied on the standard eye chart test alone. Would we tolerate such inadequate testing in other areas?

Anyone would think it preposterous that a physical exam did not include basic tests such as blood pressure and pulse rate. Yet with the exception of a handful of informed practitioners around the country, patients are rarely advised to have the special optometric testing of their vision systems even though they may have chronic unresolved learning, behavior and health problems, even though they may have consulted many practitioners without a resolution of their problems.

A growing number of psychiatrists, psychologists, pediatricians, general physicians and ophthalmologists are aware of the benefits of optometric vision therapy and do support it.

In his book, *Help for Your Learning Disabled Child*, New York psychiatrist Allan Cott, M.D., says:

> *The examination of a child who suffers from a disorder of speech, communication, or learning cannot be considered complete without a visual examination. The investigation of sight and vision is as important as any other part of the total examination--and more revealing than many other routines.*

Connecticut pediatrician Morris Wessel, M.D., reiterates this point in his book, *Raising a Healthy Child,* part of *Parents Magazine Baby and Children* series. In the foreword to Dr. Kavner's book, *Your Child's Vision,* and in other material which he has authored, including *Rickie,* a book about his daughter, Fredrich Flach, M.D., also endorses optometric vision therapy. General practitioner Dorothea Linley, M.D., of Easton, Connecticut, recommended that The *Suddenly Successful Student,* the first book on optometric vision therapy by the authors of this work, "should be part of required medical reading," particularly for physicians dealing with problem children. Ophthalmologist George Dupont, M.D., of Newport Beach, California, says that he has "been exposed to the optometric as well as the ophthalmological phases of eyecare and I refer appropriate patients. In every instance they benefit a great deal."

A valid vision analysis involves checking many different parts of the vision system. Accurate testing of schoolchildren would bring early diagnoses of those with vision imbalances. The benefits of optometric vision therapy for such youngsters would be felt in the classroom, in the community and in society at large. The difficulty up till now has been that schools have not had a comprehensive vision test. This problem has finally been resolved in the United States by the efforts of a farsighted optometric association.

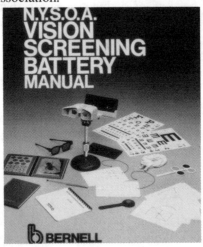

The first comprehensive vision screening battery for schools, developed through the efforts of the New York State Optometric Association.

A Valid Vision Test For Schools

The New York State Optometric Association (NYSOA) devoted quite a few years, starting in the mid-1970s, to a philanthropic endeavor: designing a comprehensive vision test to be used in schools without the help of a vision care professional. The optometrists who guided the development of this unique vision testing, Dr. Allen Cohen and Dr. Steven Lieberman, are faculty members at New York's State University College of Optometry. They received the Distinguished Achievement Award from NYSOA at its annual congress in June 1983 for this groundbreaking project. In addition to the pediatric optometrists involved in the design of the program, specialists in psychology, statistics, reading and curriculum were also part of the team.

Which States Use Comprehensive Screening?

By 1990, two states had enacted laws and guidelines for this type of school screening, Louisiana was the first, followed by New Jersey. In Louisiana, maverick citizen Charles Blaise was instrumental in working with lawmakers to develop Act No. 156 of the 1983 Regular Session of the Louisiana Legislature. The act directed each school system to implement a sensory screening program that includes visualization, audition and nutrition tests of schoolchildren's communication skills.

Sixteen independent functions of pediatric vision are checked in the test: acuity, muscle coordination, visual motor integration, eye tracking skills, convergence, color deficiency, sensory motor coordination, fusion, stereopsis, myopia, hyperopia, high astigmatism, amblyopia, binocularity and eye-hand coordination.

The distinguishing factor in the NYSOA's school vision screening test is one that will bring joy to the hearts of budget-conscious administrators. The test can be run by volunteers. A fifteen-minute audio-visual presentation offers an overview of the therapy. A brief training session prepares volunteers to give and score the test. A manual gives testing and referral details.

One of the leading manufacturers of vision therapy equipment, Bernell Corporation of South Bend, Indiana, has taken over the sales of the test equipment. Bernell, which has been in the business of serving the international community of vision care practitioners since the early 1950s, has devoted an entire page in its catalogs since 1986 to the NYSOA Battery.

Caring For the Entire Person

The professions of education and optometry have long looked at a child as a total being. The growth and development of children, as well as their reactions to and perceptions of the environment are intimately connected. Learning is work that requires a visual system capable of making many instantaneous changes and decisions about information that comes in through the visual system. The NYSOA report says, "A learner's tasks include sustained fixations, focus and eye alignment at near point, dynamic [constantly changing] focus, tracking and accommodative facility, and eye-hand coordination ability."

The report lists the requirements of a valid, reliable vision screening program:

- Clear definition of areas and skills to be screened

- Cost effective in time and money

- Clear cut referral criteria

- Efficient administration by persons with a minimum of training

- Regular retesting

What happens after testing?

It may amaze many consumers to learn that quite a few school administrators in the United States are aware of optometric vision therapy. In general, administrators have avoided the entire issue because of political ramifications. In the past, where optometrists who practice this therapy have been effective in working with the school systems, the weak point has always been referral. The burning question has been how to handle the delicate issue of referring youngsters to appropriate practitioners.

Recommendations for referral

The NYSOA project makes careful suggestions for youngsters who show vision dysfunctions. A referral letter is sent to the parents informing them that the child has been screened. If the child has not passed all parts of the screening, then the family is told which specific areas are presenting problems. A form for a vision care practitioner is also sent with the letter to the parents; this is to be completed by the practitioner. The form is specific about which parts of the test were failed: accommodation, acuity, convergence, and so on. Specific and pertinent test findings are asked for, rather than a general statement of results.

The purpose of this form is to help the screening coordinator determine whether the child has had a comprehensive examination and whether the condition identified at the screening was tested during the visual examination. It is reasonable to hope that concerned parents and a supportive school system would follow through to check that youngsters who need help to improve one or more aspects of their vision development or functioning receive help.

You will find specific guidelines for finding a good practitioner in the chapter, Help Is Here, but it can't be said too often that one of the best approaches is to telephone the practitioner and discuss the approach she or he takes and also ask for the name of a patient as a reference.

20/20 Is Not Enough

Let's consider what it means if your eyesight is described as an Olympian 20/20. The measurement simply refers to one aspect of your vision system and means you can see clearly at 20 feet what most people see clearly at 20 feet. But what about the rest of your vision system? If you see clearly, 20/20 or better--20/15, perhaps--you can still have imbalances in your vision system. If this is the case, you might function like a six-cylinder engine limping along on five cylinders, because faulty vision helps trigger faulty learning or behavior.

Dr. Richard Apell, an Associate Director of The Gesell Institute and Director of its Department of Vision for many years, explains that the vision system cannot be examined and assessed by measuring the visual clarity only. Yet the average eye exam tests for visual performance only by the ability to read letters at a distance, on an eyechart. In contrast, vision is measured in terms of actual achievement, or function, of the vision system. Six broad areas are considered:

Gross motor control
Hand-eye control

Eye control
Visual language skill
Visualization
Perceptual organization

Among the imbalances the behavioral optometrist may discover when analyzing the vision system are:

Antimetropia	one eye farsighted, the other near-sighted
Aniseikonia	each eye perceiving different size or distance;
Esophoria	overconverging of eyes, for specific distance--eyes tend to turn, what we call crossed;
Exophoria	eyes tend to slip apart, what we might call wandering or "wall" eye.

Although we can notice an eye or eyes that turn in or out, esophoria and exophoria may also be present but not visible to the onlooker. Often, these conditions can be discovered only through special testing.

How Vision Affects Learning.

Do both your eyes converge so that they aim at exactly the same place? (The technical word is fixates, which denotes spatial direction.) Does each eye make smooth, precise movements along a line of print? Most importantly, can you do both at the same time? If you do not have both of these oculomotor abilities, or cannot combine them efficiently, you will lose your place, skip lines, miss words or parts of words. As a final, bitter proof, you will have a low comprehension of the material.

Vision problems do not "cause" learning disabilities. Poor visual skills interfere with the learning process, just as a house built on sand is not secure. Good vision skills, however, provide a solid foundation for learning.

The impact of vision on learning is substantial.

Dr. Elliott B. Forrest, a leader in the field of optometric vision therapy, described in the *Journal of Optometric Vision Development* of June 1982 the intimate connection between learning and vision.

> We accept the fact that a moving vehicle may be "tracked" visually and that fixation can be shifted from a newspaper to the television set and back, with immediate single and clear vision at all distances. We take for granted that words can be visually fixated as one reads while gaining meaning from the printed symbols.
>
> We take for granted that we can look at a window display and know the feel of the material being displayed; see out of the corner of our eye while driving; light a cigarette without having to feel where the end of that cigarette is in space; solve jig-saw puzzles without having to feel and force each piece into place; and judge the height of a step or a curb as we approach it.
>
> Each of these activities requires the use of different yet interacting visual skills. Most of these skills as well as others equally as important, are directly or indirectly involved in the acts of learning and reading.
>
> An inefficiency in visually tracking consecutive words or phrases can cause a visual "stumbling" effect that could make reading to learn as well as learning to read less efficient. A poor "anticipatory" ability of the right visual field can cause problems in accurately directing the eyes to the right thus causing a tendency, when reading English from left to right, for words or parts of words to be skipped, substituted or mispronounced. An inadequate "anticipatory" ability of the left visual field can cause a tendency to miss the proper line or at least the first words in the next line as one shifts from the end of the line one is reading. Inefficiency in using two eyes as a team may result in faulty fixation skill and literally cause visual confusion as the printed page

is scanned for meaning. Accommodative (focusing) difficulties can affect the ability to sustain attention, concentrate, and process information effectively. An inability in changing focus efficiently from one point in space to another may tend to cause one to lose one's place when momentarily glancing up from the book.

It is hard to find a more concise yet eloquent analysis of the interaction of vision skills, which is why Dr. Forrest is acclaimed as one of the giants of behavioral optometry. Dr. Martin H. Birnbaum, a longtime associate of Dr. Forrest's and a major force in the field, once described Dr. Forrest as "the quintessential behavioral optometrist ... philosopher, clinician and teacher." Although he had a private practice in Long Island, New York, Dr. Forrest was also head of the Infants' Vision Clinic at the State University of New York College of Optometry for many years and a member of the college faculty. He lectured and published extensively on functional vision: how vision works. Dr. Forrest's book, *Stress and Vision,* published posthumously by the Optometric Extension Program Foundation in 1988 was written "to explore stress (general and visual) and its many ramifications--physiological, psychological and philosophical."

Chapter 4

Clues To Spotting Vision Imbalances

"Where did my child's nearsightedness come from? Did she get it from me? I started wearing glasses for the very same problem when I was in grade school."

"You don't get potatoes if you plant petunias," Dr. Forrest would often answer when asked by parents if family characteristics could be responsible for the state of their children's vision. His answer was simple but it masked the complexities of Pandora's Box.

Heredity and your parents' health play a powerful role in shaping your genes and physiology. These are the types of factors that we traditionally identify as influences on us. Behavioral optometry has added new dimensions to the definition of how vision develops and functions in the form of environmental factors, mental as well as physical. The behavior of those around you, their attitudes and perceptions impinge on you and your vision system just as the physical aspects of your environment do.

Does your family run to athletic types or bookworms driven to bring home as many class prizes in academics as possible? The family ethic--tension or a laid-back atmosphere, positive and supportive or critical, harmonious or discordant--has a significant effect on the development and functioning of the vision system.

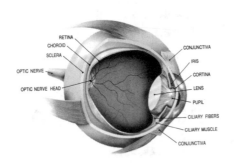

The eye, the external receptor for the vision system.

Here, we must note that a situation one person finds acceptable may well be perceived as intolerable by another. Dr. Forrest cites the analogy of the turtle and the racehorse. The turtle likes the quiet of the pond, the racehorse thrives on the hustle and bustle of the races.

An additional dimension exists: our perception of our situation. In *The Structure of Magic*, the authors explain that we each see the world differently so that each of us has a different reality. True, but consider the massive influence of a vision system which is not able to see the horizontal strokes on letters consistently. An example is the horizontal strokes in a capital *E*. Individuals with a certain type of vision imbalance will actually believe they see the letter *I* when looking at an *E*. Yes, it's possible to say that their reality is indeed different from those of us who see *E*. This is why optometric vision therapy is such a valuable, preventive health care, for it helps to bring balance to our vision systems which in turn helps our perception to be accurate.

An additional factor that influences our vision system's development is the way your family and school structure your space. Is lighting adequate, is the living space sufficient or is it cramped and crowded? How well are your basic needs filled, is furniture such as chairs and desks well designed for the individual's specific needs? The way you learn to use your time is also significant. Are the demands on your time reasonable or is there constant pressure to perform at a level that is difficult for you? Do you have enough physical exercise? Is there a heavy emphasis placed on a high level of close, academic work at an early age?

In *Stress and Vision*, Dr. Forrest is at his most eloquent. Above and beyond genetic or inherited determinants, Dr. Forrest lists the effect of developmental deprivations, one's past physical and mental history, past disease, trauma and nutritional deficiency and one's current state as contributing to the balance of one's vision system. Other factors he cites include external environmental conditions such as climate, air, water and food, pollution, crowding, and noise.

He discusses the effect on a binocular vision system geared to operate in a three-dimensional world being compelled to view flat, two-dimensional surfaces such as the television screen, video display terminal or the printed page for lengthy periods.

In a comprehensive survey of literature from many disciplines, Dr. Forrest compares the major concepts of stress and discusses their connection with vision. He suggests that individuals who are intense and analytical, who engage diligently in a task with maximum visual concentration and a strong desire for achievement while trying to get the work done as quickly as possible show a greater stress response. These are the people who are prone to stress-induced visual disorders.

The distinguished optometrist Dr. Robert Pepper of Oregon also has written of the effects of stress. Dr. Pepper, who has had great success in combining work on posture with optometric vision therapy to change visual dysfunction, has this to say in a paper, "Stress Attack, What Really Happens When One Hits," presented to a seminar at the Gesell Institute in 1985: "Under chronic stress, the kind that affects most pressured businessmen and executives day in, day out, a person is ripe for organic crisis." He also raises the question, "How does stress participate in disease? Although the intensity of the reaction varies, the sequence of events inside the body always follows the same pattern. Stress registers simultaneously in various parts of the body, including the vision system."

It's possible to improve or change many of these elements when it's discovered that they are not good for the vision of those involved, but some are inescapable because they exert themselves in the womb, in a situation over which we personally have no control.

Fetal Development

Strong influences on us before we are born are environmental factors such as drug abuse, accidents, the mother's ill health during pregnancy or a difficult birth. All these factors may harm or hinder the balanced development of the vision system in the fetus.

Those Early Weeks

In the first six months of life, the consistent development of the vision system is quite vulnerable. Dr. Torsten N. Wiesel, Chairman of the Harvard Medical School's Department of Neurobiology, one of the three researchers who shared the 1981 Nobel Prize for Medicine, did the primary study of vision development and the influence of environment. Dr. Wiesel's study showed that the development of those parts of the brain which process visual information is radically altered if the organism is deprived of adequate visual stimulation early in life and at critical periods of the developmental process. That deprivation can stem from something that is easily remedied or something that is inescapable.

For instance, early visual stimulation can be helped by attention to seemingly minor details: keeping a dim light in the nursery at night, or moving the baby's position when changing, feeding, even playing. Unavoidable happenings, such as high fever, accidents, malnutrition or severe illnesses may deprive an infant of adequate visual stimulation and disrupt the steady growth of the vision system.

A variety of childhood diseases, among them measles, influenza, encephalitis, or meningitis, can have far-reaching effects. High fever or eye or head injury in youngsters are also potential threats to young vision systems. Certain prenatal factors can put a child in the risk category of having an imbalanced vision system. They include a family history of crossed eyes, high degrees of nearsightedness or farsightedness, diabetes, sickle cell anemia, or other blood diseases. Other factors are the mother's pregnancy complications such as German measles and other viral diseases, use of drugs or toxic agents, hormonal imbalance, poor nutrition, inadequate medical care and exposure to radiation.

Most infants are born with healthy eyes and vision systems. Nevertheless, a small percentage of preschoolers have existing vision system problems. These can be the result of heredity, illness, injury or environmental factors such as lack of early visual stimulation. The fact is, the majority of vision imbalances go unrecognized until the pressures of schoolwork and study begin to overload the vision system. The sudden impact of "nearpoint" work such as reading, writing, drawing or computer use causes changes. Research also reveals that the development of a youngster's vision system is literally shaped by physical posture and constraints and the quality of mental attitudes.

The pressures of a nuclear civilization have disrupted the harmony of our visual systems. We just weren't created to handle the close work of twentieth-century technology. A tendency to nearsightedness or farsightedness will become more pronounced. An eye may begin to cross or drift. Sight may become blurred or the child may begin to see double. Most vision imbalances are triggered or aggravated by stress--often, in children, by the visual demands of schoolwork or computer use. Changes in a child's vision usually happen so gradually that a child is unaware of it. They assume that everyone sees the way they do. This can be wildly misleading to the adults in their lives because a child may have blurred vision or be seeing double and not think it worth mentioning or describing for months, even years.

Usually, the vision system is organized and functioning by the time a youngster is six. It actually takes about twelve years for the complete growth needed for us to arrive at adult vision and perception.

"I Saw Double When I Was A Child."

Double means two
that has room for

When you fold a sh

When someone says
that means you'll

Youngsters often have blurred vision but do not realize this is different from the way other people see.

The following story is the actual experience of a seven-year-old who grew up to become one of behavioral optometry's most revered practitioners, professor and writer Elliott B. Forrest, O.D., a man honored by the most prestigious awards in his field.

"One day, when I was sitting at the kitchen table after school, drinking milk and eating cookies, I looked up and saw my mother, twice. I knew I didn't have two mothers so I decided to tell my mother I saw two of her and let her handle it. I was about seven and I'd been seeing double a lot of the time, actually for as long as I could remember, but I didn't know this was different from the way anyone else saw.

"My mother was horrified and immediately called a friend. Eventually, she was given the name of an ophthalmologist on Central Park West in Manhattan. When we went to see him, he made a great impression on me. I was fascinated with the tests he made of my eyes. He discovered I had an esophoria [in-turning eye] but contrary to general practice, he did not recommend surgery but rather orthoptics." [This training, orthoptics, is used primarily to stimulate binocularity, the simultaneous use of both eyes. It has its place in therapy for the vision system but is akin to learning to drive a car through driver's education, in the school gym--a useful but limited experience.]

"As a result of the orthoptics, my double vision went away. But something else happened. I decided I wanted to help people who had problems like mine. In the next few years, I asked a lot of questions about the different types of eye care. It's amazing when I look back, I was young but I was methodical. I decided I would be an optometrist. Not an ophthalmologist, mind you, but an optometrist--one who practiced optometric vision therapy."

Dr. Forrest smiled reminiscently. As part of the research for this book, I had spent the day with him, the first of many visits either to his classes or the Infants Vision Clinic in New York City, watching as family after family brought in their youngsters. When the last group had finally departed, we had started talking about the fact that so many youngsters do not have clear vision but don't realize that blurring or doubling isn't normal. Then I had asked Dr. Forrest how he had decided to go into behavioral optometry. I had listened in delight, first to his personal story of enduring double vision as a child and then as he added a final comment.

"My family was a little puzzled when I told them my decision, but they thought it was probably a whim, like wanting to be an engine driver or a fireman. But I never changed my mind. And I have never regretted my choice."

Decades of students, patients and colleagues also have never regretted Dr. Forrest's choice of a profession. Indeed, the young boy who saw double was destined to be esteemed as a "philosopher, clinician and teacher" of towering stature.

Dr. Martin H. Birnbaum wrote in the *Journal of Optometric Vision Development* in 1986 that Dr. Forrest had a "lifelong interest in the relationship between vision and learning and established himself as a major thinker in the field of developmental vision."

When I started collaboration on the project of writing this book with Doctors Edelman and Forkiotis, one of the first recommendations made, while I was in vision therapy, was that I visit Dr. Forrest in New York. The first trip was filled with fascinating information. I kept returning to ask questions and observe Dr. Forrest with infants during the day and with doctors of optometry in residency programs, classes and clinics. On my first visit, Dr. Forrest had asked if I had read any of his work.

"I certainly have," I replied. "The first papers that Dr. Edelman gave me were your articles "Vision and the Visual Process," and "Visualization and Visual Imagery: An Overview."

"Would you like copies of my other work?" Dr. Forrest asked.

"That would be so helpful. I was heading for the library in a few minutes to see what I could find."

"Good, I will get them right now."

As I watched, Dr. Forrest moved first to one file cabinet then another, systematically pulling out article after article. He soon had a stack of journal reprints. When he handed them to me with a smile, he said, "If you have any questions about anything you read, just give me a call or come back and visit, although I am sure either of your coauthors can also help you."

On my return trips, I always had questions and Dr. Forrest always had answers. The answers might come in the form of another question, or a quiet, succinct comment, but they always came, for Dr. Forrest communicated clearly and shared his thinking openly. Dr. Birnbaum wrote, "He shared, he taught, he cared. He was interested in consciousness and in information-processing." Much of Dr. Forrest's work was devoted to those critical early years of infancy and the effect of the environment on vision.

Triggers for Vision Imbalances Dr. Forrest and many of his colleagues were concerned with the effect of posture, the quality of mental attitudes, constraints, and nearpoint work such as reading, writing and computer work on the development and functioning of the vision system. Although most of his writing is for professionals, the material is usually sparkingly clear to nonprofessionals. Dr. Forrest searched out and worked with leaders in other fields, neurology, neural anatomy, brain function, nutrition, education, psychology, and child development. Dr. Forrest is credited with major breakthroughs in the areas of imagery, visual auditory-verbal sequencing and astigmatism.

Astigmatism

This is the development of unequal curvature of the cornea. When optometrists who practice vision therapy find this type of measurement, they will commonly define it as an adaptation. In general, they believe that this type of imbalance is the result of the types of pressures mentioned above: posture, mental attitudes and so forth. Just as you might stoop to walk under a low tree branch, so you may constrict your vision system if there is a distressing level of tension in your life. If you are forced into rigid, inflexible routines, or made to sit still or focus on a book or a computer at an age when you are growing or developing and need to be flexing and moving, the end result on your particular vision system might be astigmatism.

In specific physiological terms, this means that the light gathered in by the eye is not focused properly. The consequence is blurred sight. The American Optometric Association

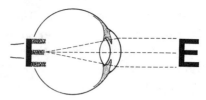

Myopic Astigmatism (Nearsightedness)

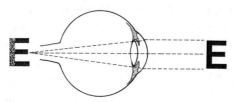

Hyperopic Astigmatism (Farsightedness)

Astigmatism comes in a variety of styles; one type means you do not see horizontal lines clearly, so a capital E might look like an I; another type of astigmatism means you have problems with vertical lines. In these cases, stairs become difficult to navigate.

(AOA) notes that only about 3 percent of school-age children have significant amounts of astigmatism; however, this represents an increase from 2 percent for preschoolers.

In 1981, in "A new model of functional astigmatism," a paper published in the *Journal of the American Optometric Association*, Dr. Forrest wrote:

Astigmatism has been of interest since Thomas Young first discovered, measured and described the condition in himself in 1801. The enigma is why it occurs. Is it mainly a structural anomaly following genetic or age trends or is it primarily functional [the way the vision system works] in nature, responding to use? Interestingly, Emile Javal, one of the early and noted researchers in the area of astigmatism, observed over a century ago that it was a common occurrence for astigmatism to decrease...after...surgery...or stereoscopic exercises (orthoptic training).

My involvement in this area was sparked by the appearance of relatively rapid and unexpected astigmatic changes in individuals of varying ages whose...status had been stable for many years.

This element of astigmatic change was investigated over a period of many years. During this time, patients...were questioned extensively and asked to demonstrate, often through the use of a visual imagery approach, how they performed their major visual tasks. This included determining how they sat, how they held their heads, and how they responded visually to secondary elements involved in their work that required looking up, down, or to the sides from what they were doing.

A subsequent research study on 45 patients showed that not only could astigmatic changes be triggered by altered eye use but that these changes could happen in as short a period as four months. A second study revealed you could analyze the data on astigmatism to predict the eye/head scan/head posture relationship.

In a paper in the December 1984 issue of the *Journal of the American Optometric Association*, "Eye scan therapy for astigmatism," Dr. Forrest reported on the results of a clinical study that involved specific eye scan therapy and its positive effects on the control and reduction of astigmatism. He and his fellow optometrists in vision therapy subscribed to the view that vision is a dynamic process. Their research and studies supported their views.

Some eye care practitioners, however, consider that astigmatism is a structural anomaly that follows genetic and age patterns. Others, notably optometrists who practice optometric vision therapy, consider that some astigmatism is a result of an interrelationship between eye scan, head scan and head posture. By changing some of these elements, astigmatism can be reduced.

Changing Astigmatism Changes Bodily Distortions Once we understand how vision imbalances such as astigmatism can develop, we can make progress in preventing or reducing them. As an indication of the intimate connection between vision and posture, astonishing changes can happen to your body when vision imbalances are helped.

One of the causes of astigmatism can be physical distortion. A child who is born with a misshapen face, or head, perhaps because of forceps delivery, might possibly have eyes that are bent out of shape also. Distortions that occur internally are usually hidden from our view, but in these cases the neurology does not develop fully or perhaps even adequately. In his book *Total Vision,* Dr. Kavner describes the case of an eighteen-month-old boy whose mother brought him in for examination.

> Johnny...held the right side of his body stiffly. His right foot turned in. When he walked he held his right hand awkwardly at his side, while the left hand swung freely.... Although his fingers were dexterous, his whole body movement was clumsy. The examination indicated that he was astigmatic in the right eye.

> Exercises were designed for him to do daily at home with his mother. These alternately used each side of his body, with his eyes steering the movements. He climbed up and down stairs and took each step with the opposite foot. He walked through a series of hoops on the floor. He crawled through a tunnel.

A few months later the astigmatism was reduced to the norm, and his body movements were coordinated. The foot no longer turned in as much.

Help From Lens Use, Also

In some cases, it is lens use which is the key factor in helping to change astigmatism. The traditional "compensating" lenses routinely prescribed are little better than crutches for the vision system. In optometric vision therapy, the lenses are prescribed either as "developmental" "stress reducing" or "remedial." The prescription of these lenses is quite different from "compensating" lenses.

You Must Want To Change

In cases of astigmatism, as in any other distortions in the vision system, the earlier optometric vision therapy is used the better. It is often easier to work with youngsters than with adults, whose warps and imbalances have been with them for many years and have thus become deeply imbedded. However, adults with astigmatism have benefited from behavioral optometry. Success is usually more likely when motivation is high.

Astigmatism Comes In Different Styles

You may have one or more types of astigmatism, such as farsighted astigmatism, or nearsighted astigmatism; also, the amount of and type of astigmatism may be different in each eye. Whatever the situation, if you have the desire to change, optometric vision therapy offers you that choice and the means.

Nearsightedness

What the eye doctor calls "myopia" is commonly called nearsightedness. Nearsighted individuals can see clearly up close but not at a distance; anything seen in the distance seems blurred. The myopic person has lost the ability to shift or relax focus and see distant objects clearly. The focus is frozen at a close distance.

Symptoms, Not Causes

In contrast to the traditional concept, which holds that the way to help myopia is to prescribe heavier and heavier compensating lenses or even to undergo surgery, behavioral optometry offers a choice, therapy to help reduce rigidity and bring some flexibility to the vision system. Optometrists who practice this therapy believe that the types of physical and mental restraints which may trigger astigmatism in some will conspire to produce nearsightedness in others. This symptom of a vision imbalance is often responsive to optometric vision therapy. By working with the cause of the vision imbalance, the symptom (nearsightedness) can be helped.

The stresses of lifestyle and environment result in visual imbalances that often end up causing rigidity in the vision system--and in mental attitudes and physical characteristics. Flexibility in the ability to make changes, whether in focusing, decision-making or physical exercise, becomes extremely difficult. Eventually, the individual sacrifices more and more flexibility. How often have you noticed that nearsighted people are detail-oriented and subjective? Usually (but not always, that is the wonderful aspect of human nature, the ability to confound the norm), it's hard for myopes to grasp concepts, to be objective. Dr. Kavner once commented that it's possible that widespread nearsightedness has been partly responsible for the conditions that led to the coining of the name "the me generation."

The Actual Figures

Probably less than 1 percent of children are born with myopia. The American Optometric Association tells us that myopia is the only refractive vision condition that increases significantly during the school years. Webster's unabridged dictionary notes that in optics, refraction is the ability of the eye to "bend" light entering it so as to form an image on the retina. To an optometrist, refraction is the clinical measurement of the eye to determine the need for lenses. Since the concepts and interpretations of measurements used by ophthalmology, general optometry and behavioral optometry differ, the definitions also differ. This is why the lenses prescribed by behavioral optometry are so different from those prescribed by other practitioners. You might say it's like comparing clothing bought off the rack to clothing made for you by a tailor who takes a wide range of comprehensive measurements of your needs. The final fit of custom clothing is personal and unique.

A Per Capita Growth

You can expect to find myopia in about 3 percent of children aged 5 to 9. It increases to 8 percent for children aged 10 to 12. Some authorities say that we are likely to find that 20 percent of an eighth grade graduating class is myopic. The right therapy can change and reduce those statistics. The Chinese have acted on their high rate of myopia. Students in China do eye exercises in class twice a day, for about ten minutes. Factory workers do, too. An official poster of eye exercises is also available. The result? A decrease in myopia in China.

Why is this? The "exercises" help bring some flexibility to the vision systems of the Chinese using these procedures. When our vision systems are less rigid and have some flexibility, we can change focus more easily and can see clearly at far as well as near distances. We will also find that our mental attitudes change, we will be more able to see other people's point of views, to change our opinions and not cling obstinately to set beliefs. Nearsightedness is a symptom of a vision imbalance that affects more than sight; treating the cause affects more than sight. Here it's important to stress one vital point that marks the difference between the traditional concepts of "eye care" and behavioral optometry.

Unfortunately, too many books and practitioners still refer to myopia as an inherited condition for which there is no known treatment. The truth is that in some cases, optometric vision therapy can reduce, even eliminate myopia in youngsters and adults.

An Epidemic Of Nearsightedness

During four years of high school, the number of nearsighted individuals increases to about 40 percent. In college, it ranges between 60 and 80 percent. In other contexts, this would be called an epidemic. The reason it has not caused alarm is that it's possible to make a myope's vision clear with prescription lenses. But lenses that only work on the symptom of near-sightedness are compensating lenses; they mask the serious nature of the condition.

Aldous Huxley, an enthusiastic supporter of optometric vision therapy, commented that the use of compensating lenses is a little like using a crutch when you have a sprained ankle. The crutch helps you move around while the ankle is still damaged. Your age and lifestyle and the extent of the damage all affect your recovery rate so, as a temporary aid, the crutch serves a useful purpose. Would you want to live with the crutch, though, for the rest of your life? Huxley compared "compensating" glasses to crutches, and said that just as one's physician would recommend physical therapy to help your body return to a decent balance, behavioral optometry prescribes a therapy for nearsightedness, in contrast to the traditional way of prescribing heavier and heavier lenses, crutches for your vision system. Optometric vision therapy offers the means to bring flexibility to the vision system and your life.

Emotional, Mental and Physical Effects of Myopia

The constraints of the vision imbalances which produce the symptom commonly described as nearsightedness have far-reaching consequences. The myopic condition literally results in body stresses that show up in our posture as well as affecting individuals mentally and emotionally. Research has shown that the metabolism of myopic people is changed. These are rarely positive, beneficial changes. Rather, they are more like the lack of flexibility that comes as we age, unless we keep active and exercise.

Another way to look at it might be to say it's like sitting in a cramped space. Blood pressure, pulses, hormones, and eventually your feelings and perceptions are all affected, rarely for the better. In war and in peace, incarceration is routinely used because of its powerful effect. The military forces have the "brig." Through the centuries, society's prisons have confined "troublemakers" in brutally restricted space. In an age when we place heavy demands on our vision, far heavier than in the past, we are neglecting basic needs and virtually incarcerating our vision systems. Optometric vision therapy can help liberate us in much the same way that physical exercise benefits us, literally expanding our horizons.

The *Philadelphia Inquirer* reported in November 1987 that almost all the markers that scientists use to measure the aging process are caused by too little exercise, rather than growing old. On the average, people over the age of 60 lose 1 percent of their muscle strength and their ability to use oxygen each year. As the ability to use oxygen diminishes, so does endurance. Yet this loss of strength and endurance can be minimized by regular exercise. A six-week program can increase thigh muscle strength in a 70-year-old by 20 percent. In four weeks, a 70-year-old can increase the ability to take in and use oxygen by 10-25 percent.

The benefits of physical exercise are well documented. From strength and endurance to lowering high blood pressure or countering obesity, even to warding off gloom and depression, walking briskly, swimming, pedaling on a stationary bicycle, all can help. Optometric vision therapy offers a similar multitude of benefits, physical and mental. The results are measurable and have been documented in research at colleges and institutions around the United States.

Behavior Affects Behavior

The environment is an integral part of the situation. A parent who is nearsighted may play a significant role in unwittingly structuring a youngster's vision system. Rigid, predictable routines with little opportunity for flexibility or options create a habitat which inevitably points the way to nearsightedness. Just as flexibility is desirable in our bodies, so, too, it is of value in our thinking and perception and behavior. Too little, or loose, structure or too much, or rigid, structure puts pressure on the vision system and brings about distortions in the way it functions and, inevitably, the way we function.

We all have seen what happens when nearsightedness strikes. Youngsters in grade school wear glasses with heavy lenses (and even if they wear contacts, the strength may be the equivalent of the thick lenses we deridingly name "coke bottle" glasses). Take a look at some of the nearsighted people around you. Are they straightbacked, do they walk upright? Do they hold their shoulders back? Many walk hunched over slightly, shoulders bent, rib cage compressed, abdomen tightened. Frequently, their gaze is on the ground, just slightly ahead of their feet. They often choose to sit close to the television set, stand close to you when talking, drive within inches of your car bumper, and hurry for the front seats in the movies. This is because their vision systems are comfortable in a small space in which they can see clearly. Since they can't see too clearly in the distance, they may ignore what lies outside the range of their vision. It doesn't take a degree in physical education to know this tight structuring will gradually affect their bodies and their behavior in less than positive ways.

What Vision Imbalances Trigger Myopia?

One young person's nearsightedness was definitely influenced by the tendency of her eyes to diverge, or break apart (an exophoria). In an effort to cope with this, her vision system responded with tighter and tighter focusing as she tried to hold both eyes straight. Poor binocularity, the simultaneous use of both eyes, also called eye teaming, may sometimes be a trigger in nearsightedness. Poor focusing ability can lead to tension in the vision system that results in myopia. The stresses of any of a variety of vision imbalances produce reactions which may lead to myopia.

The eyeball usually reaches its full size by the age of six. Yet the surge in the rate of myopia comes well after this age, often at the age of ten or eleven, when youngsters are starting to carry a heavy load academically. If you look through "compensating" glasses which have a prescription for nearsightedness, the first thing you will notice is how much smaller the lenses make objects (minification).

This brings the visual space world closer to the individual. These two factors cause the person to focus harder than normal (which brings objects close to you) and also to converge, turn your eyes in, closer than normal. As a result, peripheral space is reduced and an inwardization, or movement toward self, occurs. The tendency then may be for individuals to develop a style of "self-gratification." Perhaps they show sympathy but not empathy and find it difficult to understand the feelings and perspectives of others.

Some years ago, Dr. Forkiotis wrote that a tendency for an out-turning eye is not a cause but rather a symptom or sign of deficits in the function and performance between the two major nerve systems in the body: the autonomic and motor nerve systems. Eventually, in an effort to compensate for any vision imbalance, an individual must use an abundance of effort and energy. This use of extra effort is a drain that is like a potentially hazardous leak in the wall of a dam. Work on the leak as early as possible and difficulties can be averted.

Help to Become Flexible

Optometric vision therapy involves the use of lenses and prisms that go to the root of the myopic person's situation. Therapeutic procedures are also of value. When the correct lenses (preventive or remedial) are coupled with the correct therapy, nearsightedness may be prevented, reduced and even eliminated in some cases.

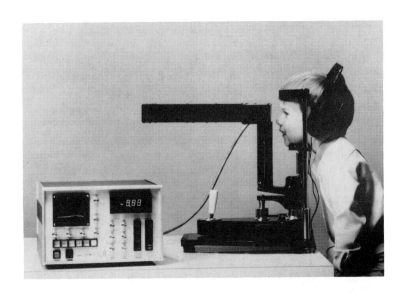

The Accommotrac equipment helps to reduce nearsightedness.

Biofeedback And Nearsightedness

Dr. Joseph N. Trachtman, a behavioral optometrist in Brooklyn Heights, New York, spent seven years developing a biofeedback device called the Accommotrac Vision Trainer (AVT). It is based on the concepts of behavioral optometry and has had a high success rate in treating nearsightedness. Patients from six to fifty-five have had good results using the AVT.

"There are no tricks or magic to it. Patients learn how to exercise and control their eye muscle, a process called accommodation," explains Dr. Trachtman. It isn't unusual for this regimen to improve a person's visual acuity, or clarity of sight. Let's say someone has 20-200 acuity, without corrective lenses; this measurement shows they can see at 20 feet what most people can see at 200 feet. The AVT can help the individual improve that acuity to 20-40, the minimum vision requirement in many states for people with corrective lenses seeking a driver's license. Of course, optometric therapy can achieve similar results without the use of the AVT. It's a little like choosing to open a can with an electric opener, convenient.

The theory behind using the ATV to help reduce nearsightedness is that if a person learns to keep the eye's ciliary muscle relaxed during focusing, substantially improved vision can result. The ciliary muscle is under the control of the autonomic nervous system. This is the system that keeps the heart beating and our lungs moving so that we breathe. One must be able to override the automatic function and begin consciously to control focusing. A key question always for the optometrist who practices vision therapy is: what is the initial cause of the myopia? This is where the exam of the entire vision system is a vital beginning point.

It's painless to use any vision training equipment, and your vision cannot be harmed. You may be given home procedures to do, though for many people good progress comes through working in the formal situation at a practitioner's office. One patient altered her nearsightedness from 20/200 to 20/40 in less than two months. Not everyone could hope to match that because her system might have had a certain degree of flexibility despite the measurement. Each individual is unique and responds differently. Dr. David Friedel of Arizona points out that it may be difficult at times to measure the success of optometric vision therapy, since the individual and the situation change constantly to meet the demands of lifestyle.

Yes, Virginia, There's Hope For Myopes

Question: The contemporary concept holds (and has held for too many decades) that the way to treat nearsightedness is to prescribe stronger and stronger lenses as one becomes more myopic. Is this concept acceptable to practitioners of optometric vision therapy?

Answer: No. These practitioners do not believe that nearsightedness is inevitable, any more than one has to endure any other vision imbalance. Rather, they feel that myopia represents a constriction in the flexibility of our perceptual, adaptive and action systems.

Whenever we have lost our flexibility, we cut back in movement and general functioning. Ultimately, lack of flexibility in the vision system can have the effect of restricting an individual's potential development.

Question: Can optometric vision therapy help reduce nearsightedness?

Answer: Yes. As with any therapy, the final results depend on the individual's motivation and general health. In the case of nearsightedness, a major influence on the quantity of change is the degree of flexibility in the various systems involved.

Question: How can optometric vision therapy help nearsightedness?

Answer: By bringing some degree of flexibility to the various systems involved. We're not talking only of physical flexibility here. Voice lessons do not train only your vocal chords. Was Vladimir Klavier Horowitz a virtuoso pianist because of his supple hands? In part, undoubtedly, but it was surely more the superb interaction of his neuromuscular, neurophysiological and neurosensory systems.

All were in harmonious integration. Since most individuals who are nearsighted have been wearing lenses from an early age, the various systems involved have grown accustomed to working in a certain way. Changes need to be made at a pace that is comfortable to the individual. There will be occasions when it is advisable not to try to make changes or to make only a certain level of changes if the myopia is deeply embedded in the individual's system.

The Proof of the Pudding

After Raymond Gottlieb graduated in 1964 with a degree in optometry, he followed a classic pattern. He taught at another college for some three years. By 1978, he had completed his

Ph.D. from the Humanistic Psychology Institute. The key departure from the traditional pattern was that Raymond Gottlieb, the optometrist, cured himself of nearsightedness in 1970. This achievement was not something that happened while Raymond Gottlieb was studying optometry. Nor did it happen while Dr. Gottlieb was teaching optometry. The transformation occurred because Dr. Gottlieb read literature that offered him options to his myopia. In his paper, "The Neuropsychology of Myopia," which appeared in the *Journal of Vision Development* in September 1980, Dr. Gottlieb says that "myopia is an adaptation to an environment which is less than healthy. ...if it is true that our ways of seeing determine what we see, what we know, and how we think, then the occurrence of myopia has important ramifications in terms of the more general problem of the effects on humans of modern civilization."

Dr. Gottlieb notes that if we are really to practice preventive health care, and to pay more than "lip service" to the idea, it's vital that there is more research to validate the concepts of behavioral optometry. As the *Review of Optometry* of May 1985 reported, the National Eye Institute was spending $41 million, or about a fourth of its budget, on research of functional vision. Other institutions and colleges of optometry are also continuing their research. Not surprisingly, since he is a practitioner and not a researcher, these days Dr. Gottlieb limits his private practice in Los Angeles to optometric vision therapy.

Reversing the Unreversible

When Robert Mucci decided to become a New York City fire fighter, he knew one thing might stop him. The city's regulations state that firemen must have uncorrected vision of at least 20/40. Mucci's was 20/400. He was nearsighted.

Omni magazine published a story, "Mending Myopia," in December 1985 explaining how, in desperation, Mucci appealed to his optometrist, Dr. Trachtman, for help. Serendipity had brought Mucci to someone well suited to the task. After twenty sessions on the Accommotrac machine developed by

Dr. Trachtman, Mucci passed the fire fighters' vision test with a score of 20/40.

These are not unique case histories. Dr. Gottlieb and Robert Mucci wanted to change their nearsightedness and were fortunate enough to find the therapy that could help. They worked on their situations and brought about improvements. Nearsightedness is often an exceptionally limiting condition, but being farsighted is not necessarily desirable, particularly if you're growing up or living in a society that places a premium on near point work (reading, writing, computer use).

Farsightedness   This is technically known as hyperopia. The American Optometric Association tells us that most schoolage children are farsighted, as nature intended them to be. As a species, our systems were admirably suited for food gathering and hunting in wide open spaces. The design of our vision system is primarily for sharp, clear seeing at a distance, the eyes of the hunter, the farmer, the sailor at sea. The effort of reading, writing, arithmetic, computer use and substantial doses of television and videos are outrages against nature.

Farsighted children can usually see well at both near and far but there is a drawback. They have to exert extra effort to bring their vision into sharp, clear focus for both near and far work. Needless to say, this is a daily stress that takes its toll.

About 6 percent of children aged five to eleven have high degrees of farsightedness and need help to relieve the tension of focusing, especially when using their eyes for close work. Most routine school eyechart exams will not catch such problems. The signs are often there, clearly visible to attentive parents and teachers. Symptoms of hyperopia include:

- Difficulty in concentrating

- Problems in keeping a clear focus when reading or doing close work

- Eye or body tension when doing such work

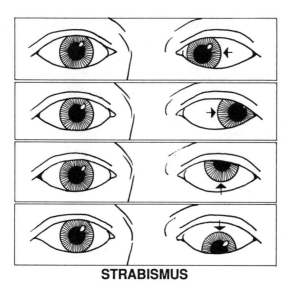

STRABISMUS

This type of visual imbalance, strabismus, is visible; most visual imbalances can only be detected by special examination.

- Muscle fatigue, headaches, nausea, or aching or burning eyes after close work

- Poor reading ability

- Irritability or nervousness after sustained close work concentration

Crossed or Out-turning Eye Let's start out by emphasizing it's never too late to try to help strabismus, an eye that turns in, out, up or down. While not common, this condition puts particular pressures on the individual who suffers from it.

The medical approach tends to blame poor eye control on the muscles of the eye and all too frequently advises surgery to alter the length of the muscles. Behavioral optometry believes differently and has a less radical, more promising approach than surgery: therapy and lens use. Since the cause of strabismus is at the cortical level (in the brain), cutting the eye muscles is rarely of benefit, other than in the rare cases of paralysis or partial paralysis of the muscles. Strabismus is a condition in which the two eyes do not work together. The causes vary. Illness, accidents or stress are factors, so is heredity. When someone has strabismus, it means that the vision system has not learned to make the two eyes work together as a team.

It is normal during the first five or six months for an infant's eyes to appear crossed or unaligned for brief moments while the baby learns to use the eyes together as a team. If, by the age of three months, the misalignment appears to be frequent or long-lasting, or is always with the same eye, an examination will reveal the extent of the problem. Crossed eyes can also develop at a later stage, as children reach school age. Oddly enough, the development is often so gradual that parents fail to recognize it. They get used to the child's appearance and it seems normal. In this case, the problem may be noticed first by the family doctor or at school.

A Cosmetic and Functional Problem   Two major factors are involved in crossed eyes. The first, and the most obvious, is appearance. Crossed eyes look funny, peculiar, different. This is the last thing anyone, young or old, wants. This "difference" can inhibit an individual's emotional and social development. It can also lead to personality problems by isolating the person from others and causing a poor self-image. The second, poor physical functioning, occurs because the eyes do not work together as a team.

The writer of this book, Hazel Dawkins, developed an in-turning eye, perhaps as a result of a high fever which occurred when she was an infant. At the age of seven, she had surgery to "straighten" the eye. Within months, the eye was turning out and Hazel could not see with it. For the next forty years, she was legally blind in that one eye. This is not unusual, and the question is, why does this happen? Surgery on eye muscles is performed in an effort to change the eye's position. It is not successful because these muscles do not control eye movement, the muscles direct movement.

The Brain Controls Eye Movement

As a youngster, before and after the surgery, Hazel was labeled clumsy. She walked into people and objects because before and after the surgery her brain had two different messages coming in through the vision system. One eye had one perspective, the other eye had another perspective. Hazel saw two doorways, two trees, two chairs, and didn't always choose the right one to navigate. Eventually, after the surgery, her brain made an executive decision. It shut down input from the strabismic eye. That was why it was not possible for her to see anything with it.

Imagine her surprise forty years later when Dr. Edelman told her she was not blind. The legal definition of blind is 20/200. Hazel's strabismic eye measured 20/400. Despite this, Dr. Edelman told her there was a distinct possibility that she could learn to straighten her eye and recover some of the lost sight and vision, without surgery. That was not all. As the therapy progressed, Hazel and her family realized there were other benefits. Her energy level increased, her balance and coordination grew better, her disposition improved, travel sickness became a problem of the past, she slept more soundly. Hazel's perception of events also changed and became more balanced as her vision system became more balanced.

In some cases, a strabismic eye may seem to straighten itself, but what actually happens is that the individual's brain shuts down the faulty receptor, the eye. In that case, although both eyes may seem to work together, they do not. Perhaps now and then both eyes work in tandem, intermittently, but that also poses problems. The individual will have physical and emotional problems that are triggered by the vision imbalance. Poor coordination, poor memory, poor recall, low self-image and lack of confidence.

Occasionally, the reverse will be found, and the individual will have a tendency toward a "superiority complex," which will make them seem arrogant. They might even turn into perpetual complainers, always making excuses at how hard their lives are, which isn't far from the truth. This is how visual imbalances create perceptual imbalances. Lack of or poor binocularity usually creates a hazardous situation for the individual physically and emotionally. Sometimes, the brain shuts down the input from one eye completely. In other cases, the brain alternates the use of first one eye, then the other. If the alternation is fast, it creates a great deal of confusion. Even when it is not fast, the individual usually finds it very difficult to handle school work and social situations. In some cases, they are set on a path which is particularly difficult to travel. For some it may lead to failure, perhaps even juvenile delinquency.

Crossed Eyes Are Not Outgrown

Parents who seek help as soon as they spot the symptoms are acting wisely. To repeat an early comment, it's never too late to try. Adults with in- or out-turning eyes have benefited from optometric vision therapy. The procedures will vary, of course, depending on the needs of the patient. One of the most useful pieces of equipment used to stimulate binocularity are glasses with one red and one green lens (the lens has no prescription). The patient wears the red and green glasses and looks at a chart or other equipment that is also part red and part green. The red filter in the glasses will neutralize the green on the chart, and the red on the chart will be neutralized by the green filter in the glasses.

Unless both eyes are used, a total picture of the chart cannot be seen when the red-green glasses are worn. If one eye is not teaming with the other, part of the chart will seem blank. As the eyes learn to work with each other, the patient will be able to see all of the chart through the red-green glasses. Once this is a consistent response, the individual is clearly using both eyes and teaming them. In all likelihood, behavioral changes will also occur.

In the 1986 publication, "*Vision Therapy and Insurance: A Position Statement,*" from the State University of New York State College of Optometry, two important papers are published in appendices xiii and xiv: the first, "Orthoptic Treatment of Strabismus," by Nathan Flax, M.S., O.D., and Robert Duckman, M.A., O.D., and the second, "Results of Surgical Treatment of Intermittent Divergent Strabismus," by Dr. Flax and Arkady Selenow, O.D. Readers who would like more information on strabismus will find these papers, which are carefully documented, of great value. The college's address appears in the back of this book if your local resources do not include the publication.

Lazy Eye   Amblyopia is often called "lazy eye," and it is a condition in which clear, sharp vision in one eye is lowered or apparently lost and cannot be improved with prescription "compensating" lenses. It affects about 2 percent of the population. The American Optometric Association tells us that there are different kinds of lazy eye. The most common type is a side effect or complication stemming from strabismus or from a vision condition in which one eye is much more nearsighted or farsighted than the other. In either of those situations, the two eyes send separate and different messages to the brain, which cannot integrate them. Therefore, the brain often turns off the message from one eye. Since the ability to see sharply and clearly is a learned skill, central visual acuity does not develop properly in the eye the brain turns off. The one-eyed or partial vision that invariably results can affect other skills, such as the ability to judge distances, although someone with a lazy eye will not realize this.

Behavioral optometry believes that near- and far-sightedness and astigmatism are adaptations made by individuals to help them perform adequately. The need for such adaptations may be alleviated when the entire vision system is working smoothly.

Clues are head tilting, which usually means one eye is being favored, and a tendency to bump into objects. Since poor vision in one eye does not necessarily mean amblyopia, or "lazy eye" (it could mean nearsightedness), amblyopia can only be definitely diagnosed by a professional examination. Remember that often the lazy-eyed individual becomes one sided in responses and movements and usually does not develop the concept of opposites. Perhaps there is difficulty in balancing or sports. Sometimes, certain activities like dancing that require using two sides of the body may be avoided.

Chapter 5

The Problems Are Legion

The kind of vision-related learning, behavior or health problems we're discussing in this book probably will not be uncovered in the typical Snellen eyechart exam. Nor will an exam that is limited to checking eye health and acuity (clarity of sight) expose vision dysfunction. Naturally, if you've had a basic exam of this type (before you had learned there's another type of exam) and had been given a clean bill of health by an eye care professional, you will believe, reasonably so, that any learning, behavior or health problems you might be experiencing stem from causes in other parts of your body or mind, not from your eyes. Logically, the exam was accurate. But although you might have excellent eye health and acuity, the test had not covered your complete vision system.

The crux of the matter is that it's often virtually impossible to know it's your vision system that isn't working smoothly when you have symptoms of vision dysfunction. Sprain your ankle and you know what you've done. It's fairly hard to mistake toothaches. But vision dysfunction is somewhat like static or interference on the television screen. The actual problem may be elsewhere. It may be in the television set, it may be in the transmittal, or the source of the program might be the culprit. So it is with our vision systems.

Potential sites for vision problems are in the transmittal route (the optic pathway) or the program source (the visual cortex, the back part of the brain). Warps, imbalances, developmental lags in the vision system, or immaturity of the system, may be responsible for snarls that result in disruptions to learning, behavior or health. Occasionally, paralysis of the muscles that move the eyes is the cause of vision problems. And when we don't know how to read the clues, or symptoms, of vision dysfunction, it's easy to mislabel them. At one end of the scale, youngsters with undiagnosed vision dysfunction have been mistakenly labeled dyslexic, delinquent and learning disabled. At the other end, adults have been wrongly identified as chronic schizophrenics, alcoholics or severely depressed.

These grave errors spring from several sources: society's need to put us in categories and the consumers' lack of knowledge of and information about behavioral optometry and optometric vision therapy. The individuals in the following case histories were chronic psychiatric patients. Their conditions were "chronic" because they were of six or more months' duration. The patients had been given quality care by dedicated health professionals at top-level institutions. The flaw was the lack of knowledge about a therapy which had the potential to help.

More than half (66 percent) of the people in a seven-year study had "significant impairments in visual-perceptual function." The study paper, "Visual Perceptual Dysfunction in Psychiatric Patients," by Frederic F. Flach, M.D., and Melvin Kaplan, O.D., appeared in *Contemporary Psychiatry* of July-August 1983 and was also incorporated in the continuing medical education materials, *Directions in Psychiatry*, volume 3, lesson 10, and in educational material published by the Optometric Extension Program Foundation. Psychiatrist Dr. Flach is Adjunct Professor of Psychiatry at Cornell University Medical College and

Attending Psychiatrist at the Payne Whitney Clinic of the New York Hospital and St. Vincent's Hospital and Medical Center of New York. Behavioral optometrist Dr. Kaplan is a Fellow of the College of Optometrists in Vision Development; Instructor, Department of Psychology at Mercy College, Dobbs Ferry, New York; and a member of the New York State Board of Examiners in Visual Training. In 1990, the book *Rickie* by Flach and his daughter was published. It is the poignant history of the daughter's struggle with what was mistakenly labeled and treated as schizophrenia but which turned out to be abnormal behavior triggered by vision imbalances. Optometric vision therapy helped Dr. Flach's daughter overcome the abnormal behavior, leave the institution and live a normal life.

Schizophrenia Subdued

A twenty four-year-old woman, whom we'll call Bernadette, had spent close to ten years in and out of psychiatric hospitals. She had had episodes of depression and acute psychotic behavior. Labeled schizophrenic, just about every type of psychological therapy and psychiatric drug had been tried on Bernadette without any discernible result. She was not able to attend school or do part-time work and had virtually withdrawn from social contacts. Equally sad was the fact that Bernadette was convinced of her incurability. Her family and Dr. Flach, her psychiatrist, had finally concluded that they had exhausted all possible avenues of hope. Schizophrenia is a notoriously difficult condition. Bernadette was one of those notoriously difficult schizophrenics. Then came her first visual examination by behavioral optometrist Dr. Kaplan.

Bernadette told Dr. Kaplan she had difficulty reading. She also said that visual images rarely lasted more than a minute or so and that she could keep her vision for longer periods only with great effort of will. When asked if she could remember when this problem had first begun, she recalled that it went back to when she was four. Bernadette had been looking out of her bedroom window and had seen the trees and bushes moving in toward her. She was terrified. She also remembered that a few hours before this, she had been very frightened at overhearing an argument between her parents in the next room. Since the age of thirteen, every attempt to do her schoolwork had left Bernadette in great confusion, often to the point of disorganizing panic. This led to her being in and out of institutions and gradually being forced out of the mainstream of life by her apparent schizophrenia.

Dr. Kaplan's examination revealed a high level of spatial orientation dysfunction (difficulty knowing the accurate position of anything at which she looked). Bernadette's reaction to the testing showed how her vision system behaved under stress. She had hysterical amblyopia (diminished vision) that measured 20/200--the measurement of those legally blind. During the test, her eye movement control became very erratic and she had difficulty changing focus so that she could see clearly at near point (a book, for instance). She also stopped using much of her peripheral vision and showed a mostly central vision.

The conclusion of Dr. Kaplan's exam was that although Bernadette's visual system was essentially free of disease, she was for all practical purposes functionally blind--her vision system functioned like that of a nearly blind person. Bernadette, a chronic schizophrenic patient, had certainly had her eyes examined before. She had certainly reacted in the same way. The trouble was that during her previous exams, eye health and acuity (clarity of sight) had been checked, nothing more! Bernadette had not been examined before by a practitioner of optometric vision therapy.

How Was Bernadette Helped?

Dr. Kaplan's treatment for Bernadette combined optometric vision therapy and constant use of vertical yoked prisms. This type of prism is essentially prisms of equal degree, with both bases placed in the same direction. For people whose vision system is centrally organized, the bases are placed down. People who are peripherally organized benefit from bases placed up. The purpose of this is to introduce flexibility into the visual-perceptual system so that the individual can adapt to changing situations and learn, step by step, how to see and understand what is happening.

A positive change for Bernadette was not long in coming. By the end of the first six weeks, her posture and dress improved. She did not walk slumped over, peering at the floor, as she had been doing for so long. By the end of the first twelve weeks, she was able to pass the test for a driving license and she began to drive a car. Within six months she was discharged from the hospital. She was able to go to college and eventually graduate. Her life became thoroughly normal.

In the years following Bernadette's optometric vision therapy in the late 1970s, she has not shown any symptoms of schizophrenia. Not only has Bernadette been able to leave the psychiatric institution, she has successfully created an independent life for herself. College, a job, marriage, motherhood. This was Bernadette's accomplishment. A far cry from the twenty-four-year-old who had spent almost a decade in and out of psychiatric hospitals, struggling to overcome an illness misdiagnosed as psychiatric.

Not A Cure-all

Not all schizophrenics have vision-perceptual disorders. It is regretfully true that Dr. Kaplan, Dr. Flach and their colleagues will not be able to rid us entirely of schizophrenia. But for those psychiatric patients whose vision dysfunction is triggering their abnormal behavior, and whose physicians know about behavioral optometry, the potential for dramatic, beneficial change exists.

Depression Overcome

Anna was thirty-two and single when she went to see psychiatrist Dr. Frederick Flach. She said she had been having persistent feelings of depression which seemed very strong during the year before her first visit. Later, she described herself as having been depressed since her mid-teens. One of Anna's problems was difficulty falling asleep at night, and now and then she also went through phases of waking up early in the morning. Her sexual desire suffered, she found it extremely hard to concentrate on work and she had an aversion to seeing friends or family. Her self-confidence was so poor she was convinced she would lose her excellent job as assistant marketing director for a large magazine.

An unhappy love affair and a job promotion seemed to have been reasons for the intensifying of her depression about a year before the first consultation. For nearly eight years, Anna had been dating and then had lived with a divorced man ten years her senior. Although she felt she loved this man, to whom she had become intensely attached, she did not receive any commitment of marriage from him. Her promotion had been something of a burden. She had been in a sales job which she had handled well and found satisfying. In the old job, Anna was out working in the field, while the new job kept her in the office and also demanded a far more structured day.

Anna was not the first in her family to have difficulty coping. Her mother and one of her siblings had suffered with depression. Her father had been killed in a car crash when Anna was six and she had no memories of him. Although she was ambitious and eager to succeed academically, it had often been a struggle for Anna to do well and to make a good career for herself.

In the first three months of individual psychotherapy, Anna showed some improvement. She was put on an antidepressant drug, maprotiline, after the first month of therapy. This was something Anna accepted with reluctance, for she had hoped to avoid drugs. While the drug did help the depression, some of the other major difficulties, such as her inability to concentrate and her low self-esteem about her abilities at work persisted and were almost crippling. Anna lived in fear that her boss would fire her because she had such difficulty in focusing on her work and constantly procrastinated.

A recommendation was made by Dr. Flach for the second time that Anna have a visual-perceptual analysis. This time she accepted, although reluctantly. The exam by Dr. Kaplan showed that Anna had quite severe vision imbalances. She had difficulty coordinating her eyes and concentrating on objects and people close at hand; she also had poor focusing abilities. And because her system chose to narrow itself from three-dimension vision to two-dimension vision at times, she suffered from inconsistent perceptual vision, which made it hard for her to be spatially organized.

How Was Anna Helped?

Dr. Kaplan prescribed home procedures that were designed to bring some balance to the problem areas in Anna's vision system. She also had a special pair of prisms to wear at all times, except when driving at night. The prisms have the effect of starting visual-perceptual change by compression and expansion of space and the direction of objects at which you look.

Anna noticed changes within several weeks. She felt less pressured at work. Gradually, over the next few months her work ability grew and her productivity increased. She did not find it hard to focus on her work and she did not procrastinate. By the end of six months, she did not have to wear the prisms any longer.

Optometric vision therapy helped Anna overcome depression which had been with her every day for more than half her life. It had harmed her personal relationships and threatened her career. Until her psychiatrist was able to persuade her to add optometric vision therapy to counseling, the progress in fighting Anna's depression was limited and had little hope of making any meaningful changes. Optometric vision therapy was a successful and swift treatment.

Help For Psychiatric Patients

In the conclusion to their article, "Visual-Perceptual Dysfunction in Psychiatric Patients," Dr. Flach and Dr.Kaplan wrote:

It would seem that there is definitely a relationship between certain psychiatric disorders and visual-perceptual dysfunction, particularly among patients diagnosed as having schizophrenic disorders, recurrent unipolar depression, and alcoholism. Chronicity of illness (in excess of six months) and social withdrawal or occupational difficulties seem to be most marked among such patients.

Although the exact nature of the relationship between dysfunction and psychopathology remains unclear, the fact that the presence or absence of such dysfunction can be so easily determined should make us consider visual-perceptual analysis as a routine procedure in the evaluation of all psychiatric patients. Moreover, by means of visual training, the ability of such patients to function may often be substantially enhanced.

Chronic Health Problems

Undiagnosed vision problems precipitate a host of health difficulties. Migraines, headaches, muscle aches, back and neck pain, sleeplessness, bed-wetting, travel sickness, dizziness, teeth grinding, allergies--the list is lengthy. A major signal that a problem might be stemming from the vision system is when individuals have trekked from clinic to clinic, or practitioner to practitioner, searching fruitlessly for help. Then it's time to suspect that the vision system might be triggering health problems that haven't responded to traditional health care for the simple reason that the source of the trouble hasn't been diagnosed and treated.

Rosa Woodston and Becky Allerby are two people who had suffered from debilitating migraines most of their lives. Rosa was in her seventies by the time she found optometric vision therapy. Becky was more fortunate, she was ten years old when her mother took her to Dr. Edelman. Each had sought help from a wide range of health care practitioners. Each had had their eyes checked regularly and been given clean bills of health, although it's significant to note that neither had been examined by a behavioral optometrist.

Home Tutoring The Only Answer?

By third grade, Becky Allberby's parents decided to keep their daughter home from school and give her home tutoring.

"The teachers couldn't have tried harder," said Becky's mother. "They went beyond the call of duty but Becky just couldn't learn. We all knew she had some sort of learning problem, for she tried hard and was never in trouble for her behavior. The school offered all sorts of remedial education, but finally we decided that it would be easier on everyone if we worked at home. At first, it did seem to help. The pressure of trying to keep up with a classful of her peers was off Becky and she still had plenty of friends in the neighborhood and at church. But then, after the first year she was home, she started having severe migraines.

"For about a year, which was when she was nine, the migraines only hit now and then. By the time she was ten, they were fairly regular. They just about immobilized her. Some days it would be so bad, she'd be flat on her back from noon on. I'd read to her, do some problems aloud, but I felt she was falling behind in her education.

"Our own relationship was being strained because sometimes I thought she was faking, and, of course, she could tell what I was thinking. Eventually, our family doctor said there was nothing left to do but take Becky to a neurologist. He'd exhausted his possibilities. We were so worried. The obvious thought was a brain tumor. I talked to my minister about my fears, and he suggested that before I go to the neurologist I consider taking Becky to Dr. Edelman. Purely as a way of avoiding the neurologist, we went to Dr. Edelman, although I had no real hope.

"The exam Dr. Edelman gave Becky was totally different from any eye exam she'd ever had before. At one point, we watched Becky through a one-way mirror, to see how she worked on some drawing she'd been given to do. As we watched, she turned the paper completely around in order to draw a horizontal line, in effect drawing a vertical line instead. She often did the same thing when doing her work. As Dr. Edelman tested Becky, it was clear even to me that her visual abilities were not at all good.

"Dr. Edelman said that he thought he could help. He loaned me a pair of glasses. Stress-reducing lenses, he said. He asked me to call in two days. 'I think you will have some good news for me,' he said. 'I believe Becky's vision imbalances are the cause of her migraines. These lenses should go a long way toward changing the situation.'" Mrs. Allerby smiled as she recollected that day at Dr. Edelman's office.

"I remember staring at Dr. Edelman in amazement. All I could think was how could he possibly be right? Becky's eyes had been checked quite a few times before, although the previous exams had taken just a few minutes and no one had ever done the sort of tests this doctor had. So I decided it was worth a try. We went home, with Becky wearing the glasses.

"Forty-eight hours later, I called Dr. Edelman to tell him that he was right. Becky hadn't had a migraine since we'd left his office. That was wonderful. Something else had happened that was also important. Up to then, she'd been able to work only for about fifteen minutes before a blinding migraine would hit. Since she'd been wearing the glasses, she'd worked for nearly two hours before we'd stopped only because she was tired."

Becky has not had a migraine since her first visit to Dr. Edelman in December 1985. As a further grace note, Becky had always been prone to travel sickness and headaches. She does not have either any more. Becky has also been able to accomplish her dearest wish--to join her friends at school. In January, she started taking regular vision therapy from Dr. Edelman. In the summer, she went to a local learning center for professional tutoring so that she could enter school in the fall, on grade level for her age.

Migraines For Fifty Years

Rosa Woodston arrived in the United States from her native Switzerland in the 1930s when she was in her early twenties. Her husband taught theology at Villanova University. They lived in the pleasant suburbs outside Philadelphia, where they raised their son. Rosa's migraines had started at about the time she arrived in America. Nothing helped. She tried everything her physician and the hospital had suggested, including a wide variety of medication. Despite all their attempts, several times a month Rosa would have to stay in bed for a few days to "wait out" the crippling effects of the migraine.

"It was impossible to plan anything with any certainty," she explains. "I'd always say, if I can be there I will, but I may be incapacitated."

A member of the Quaker meeting in Radnor, Pennsylvania, the Religious Society of Friends, which the Woodstons had attended for many years, knowing of the connection between vision and migraines showed them the paperback, *Suddenly Successful Student.*

"I know you've tried everything possible for your migraines, Rosa. Perhaps this optometrist could help?"

"Isn't this interesting?" Rosa said to her husband. "You know, I've worn glasses since I was seventeen and they've never really been right."

When the Woodstons visited Dr. Edelman, he was able to make the same prediction for Rosa that he had for Becky.

"Your vision system's imbalances are undoubtedly triggering your migraines. The lenses you have now are not right for your vision needs. Here's a prescription for different lenses."

Rosa's migraines were not quite the same to resolve as Becky's. Rosa's problem had existed for more than fifty years, whereas Becky had suffered for about three years. But within two months of wearing the correct lenses, Rosa's migraines had been reduced by 90 percent. Within six months, they had virtually disappeared.

"This has really changed the quality of my life," says Rosa. "Needless to say, I feel much more relaxed since I know that a migraine isn't hovering. I don't have to take strong medication since I don't have the migraines anymore. My husband and I are able to plan our days without wondering if we will have to cancel something.

"Our families in Europe were very interested in the news," Rosa adds. "Particularly our son. He had had learning difficulties as a youngster. He made inquiries and found an optometrist who practices this specialty near where he lives in Switzerland. Now he also has different glasses and is much more comfortable."

Headaches And Claustrophobia

Glenn Thompson grunted in satisfaction as his baseball bat connected with the ball. It was a homer to left field. Behind him, his teammates on the semi-pro Tigers yelled their approval.

"You're predictable, thank the lord," his coach called out approvingly, as Glenn jogged home past third base. "Darned if I've ever seen you hit anywhere else--but if that's your sweet spot, hey, I'm all for it."

Glenn smiled in agreement. He did always hit to left field, but with a batting average of .450 he was a valued player for two semi-pro teams when the season was in. He nodded his head at the coach and then instantly regretted it, he could feel a headache starting. One of the reasons he played ball was to try and reduce stress and tension. It didn't seem to help that much, nor did going to the gym three or four times a week on his lunch hour, either playing paddle ball or working with weights. His headaches seemed as regular as his routine.

Glenn, a financial planning and insurance advisor with a large company, saw clients at their homes in the evening, after a six-hour day at the office. In the past few years, he had deliberately reduced his travel schedule because of an increasing intolerance for flying and crowds. Glenn literally became claustrophobic on airplanes. Yet he had served in the US Navy aboard an aircraft carrier, on the flight deck. He had not been particularly uncomfortable in the limited space, although his headaches had been severe. Glenn could remember being plagued by headaches since he was about eight years old. He had visited many specialists and had been given a wide range of tests, but always their conclusion was that no specific reason could be found for his headaches, which for some reason were more severe on weekends.

"Will contact lenses help me?"

Glenn was twenty-six years old when he made an appointment with Dr. Forkiotis to discuss the possibility of having contact lenses.

"I'd like contacts for cosmetic purposes and I'm wondering if they might help with my problems, like the headaches and claustrophobia," Glenn said to Dr. Forkiotis at the beginning of the vision analysis.

"It's three years since my last eye exam with a practitioner in another town. I wear my glasses all the time. I was told they are very weak, and I only have to wear them when I feel the need but I feel they might help, so I tend to wear them all the time."

"How much reading do you do?"

"A great deal. I have to keep up with the technical journals, but I also read for pleasure. Any spare moment I have I'm reading, either for business or general interest."

"Apart from what you've already told me about fairly regular headaches and growing claustrophobia, are there any other health problems?"

"Not really. Well, there's one thing--I have a yearly physical and I always faint during the exam."

"Really? What does your physician say about this?" Dr. Forkiotis asked.

"He says I'm not to worry about it, since it doesn't hamper the exam."

When Dr. Forkiotis had finished the vision exam, he took the time to explain the results.

"Your clarity of sight is 20/25, and at close work you are capable of 20/20 with each eye and with both eyes working together. However, the findings indicate that your focusing ability does not function well and you are not able to keep your focus efficiently for any length of time. As a consequence of constantly forcing your vision system to try to focus, you literally end up with headaches. Inevitably, this in turn increases the severity of the perceptual problems. Regretfully, the lenses you were prescribed before you came to me compound the symptoms."

Glenn listened in astonishment.

"Is there anything you can do?"

Solutions That Work

"Certainly. I am going to prescribe lenses for close work. They will help to relieve your general physical and visual stress by balancing the convergence-divergence and focus mechanisms. I suggest you consider coming to my office for therapy, so that you can learn how to improve the way your vision system functions. I will develop a program of home procedures for you to do, also."

Glenn started wearing the different prescription Dr. Forkiotis had recommended. He found that his headaches were greatly reduced. Reading was much more comfortable. Office visits, once a week for an hour, began and so did home procedures, which were to be done at least five times a week, for fifteen to twenty minutes.

Excellent Results

After eleven sessions, Glenn's headaches were gone, completely. He also lost his claustrophobia. Travel by plane became comfortable and posed no problems. His batting average remained high, but now Glenn was aware of the right field. He found he could hit the ball where he chose to direct the hit. During therapy with Dr. Forkiotis, Glenn had become aware that he was suppressing the right visual field. This had affected many of his daily visual tasks and his baseball and had contributed greatly to much of his general physical stress.

Glenn began to think back to the days before he'd started the therapy. He began to understand why he had had to sit in certain positions, inevitably choosing an open area for his left side. If he had to be next to a wall or any large object on the left, he felt very uncomfortable. Other benefits became apparent. Glenn was able to organize his time more profitably. He stopped playing baseball so that he could spend more time with his wife. Since he still worked out at the gym at lunch time, he wasn't missing the exercise, he just didn't need to try to get out more because of headaches and tension. Eventually, Glenn opened his own financial management business. He visits Dr. Forkiotis regularly to make sure that the stress-relieving lenses are still appropriate; the prognosis is that the lenses will provide enhancement of Glenn's visual performance for years to come.

Muscle Aches And More

How is it possible to link that nagging backache or sore neck to your eyes? Remember that your eyes are the end receptors of a system that relays a great deal of information to your brain and your body. The statistics are staggering: each eye has one billion nerve fibers that feed the brain. The brain processes three billion impulses every millisecond: one billion from each eye and one billion impulses from the rest of the body. The link between muscle aches and those nagging problems like travel sickness or teeth grinding is the fact that 20 percent of the nerve fibers of the retina go to the neck and back. Out of the billions of impulses traveling through the vision system, 20 percent directly affect the neck and back.

This means that your vision system affects your posture--and posture affects your vision system. Warps, gaps or lags at any point in the vision system will distort the neurological impulses going to the neck and back. Usually, such distortions lead to muscle tension. From there, the route to chronic aches is swift. If you've ever sprained, dislocated or broken anything, you are well aware that the body will share the work of the damaged part. One actually can strain other parts of the body trying to manage without, say, full use of an ankle. Even if this doesn't happen, you build up a lot of tension in other areas while the damaged part is mending.

This writer suffered for years from neck and back pain which, although relatively minor, was impossible to lose. Exercise helped, so did shiatsu but inevitably the tightness and soreness crept back. It was quite a surprise to realize that these aches had disappeared within a few months of taking optometric vision therapy and wearing lenses prescribed by Dr. Edelman. Another delightful loss was travel sickness, which for years had made journeys a daunting prospect, particularly those by car. It's uncanny to be abandoned by those longtime companions, particularly since they were not the reason for going to Dr. Edelman in the first place. For many, however, such difficulties are clues, especially when chronic muscle ache, dizziness, teeth grinding, bed wetting, claustrophobia or travel sickness have not responded to other help.

Learning Disabilities

This area is a cruel swampland which traps too many youngsters. If not corrected, their dysfunctions will be with them for the rest of their lives. The number of labels for those unable to perform either at their potential or at the norm for their age grows like topsy. Parents and teachers are all too familiar with the list--they also know the youngsters who have difficulty in the general classroom and who haven't benefited greatly from the special education courses or remedial education. These problems rarely lessen with age. New York psychiatrist, Dr. Allan Cott says,

A learning-disabled child grows up to be a learning-disabled adult.

In the United States, the legal definition is that a learning disability is present when a child is two years or more behind in reading and writing. In the *New York Times* of November 11, 1984, the number of students in the United States diagnosed as learning disabled was given as 1.8 million. Those are the youngsters in school who clearly fall within the boundaries of the legal definition of learning disabled, but as any educator will tell you, the actual number of children who struggle ineffectually to learn is far higher. In his book, *Help for Your Learning-Disabled Child*, Dr. Cott says: "Learning disabilities constitute the most prevalent and urgent medical problem of children in the developed countries of the world." He estimates that in the United States alone there may be some 10 million youngsters whose learning functions are impaired and whose disorders range from mild to thoroughly incapacitating.

Optometric vision therapy is not going to rid us of learning disabilities. But it has helped a high proportion of youngsters and adults labeled learning disabled. This therapy is of value when vision imbalances are triggering the learning difficulties.

Superior Abilities But Learning Disabled

Over the years, the professional magazine, *Optometry Times*, has featured a column, "My Most Interesting Case," sponsored by Marchon Eyewear, Inc. The August 1984 issue carried a case study by Dr. Beth Bazin, who was at that time assistant clinical instructor and a member of the residency program for behavioral optometry at the State University of New York College of Optometry. Before becoming an optometrist, Dr.

Bazin had been an educator who specialized in working with learning disabled children.

"When I was teaching, my mentors were two inspiring women who had long recognized the value of optometric vision therapy for children with learning difficulties. Eventually, I decided that I would make a drastic career switch, leave my job, take a loan and go back to college--this time for a degree in optometry and then continue on to a residency in behavioral optometry," Dr. Bazin explained.

In the column she writes that "K.M. wins the honor of my most interesting case not because his case was unique, but because I taught K.M. one summer in a school for the learning disabled and three years later was able to evaluate his progress after optometric vision therapy."

It is rare for someone who has the professional qualifications in both education and behavioral optometry to have the opportunity to work with a youngster after an interval of several years. After he completed third grade, K.M. had spent the summer of 1980 at the Churchill School. His performance was average in a group of seven. A shy child, he rarely volunteered answers. He had been classified learning disabled on the basis of tests administered in the spring of 1980. On the Wechsler Intelligence Scale (revised), K.M. had a verbal IQ of 119, a performance IQ of 130 and a full-scale IQ of 127. The Bender-Gestalt revealed an age equivalent of 10-10 to 10-11 (chronological age 8-8). His oral reading and listening comprehension were at the third grade level and silent reading was at the second-grade level.

Other tests showed normal skills. His overall cognitive abilities were in the superior range, but difficulties were noted in the areas of visual and auditory perception and visual perception and memory. Handwriting skills and written expression were below the level expected and there were problems with written spelling. K.M. was unable to keep up with his classwork. He was well behaved in class but lacked confidence. When Dr. Bazin gave K.M. an optometric exam, the 21-point evaluation of the vision system and other types of behavioral optometric tests showed responses below that normally expected and of an inconsistent level. K.M. reported he often found words blurring, he had double vision, the printed letters "floated," and he lost his place when reading. The optometric diagnosis was accommodative and convergence infacility. This meant that K.M. had difficulty changing focus to see clearly at different distances, as well as problems with his eyes working as a team when he used them for close work. Suddenly, the puzzle of how a youngster with K.M.'s superior abilities is performing poorly has some answers.

Dr. Bazin began vision training for K.M. that June. She also prescribed lenses for him to use while reading. The program was designed to develop ease of the accommodative response and to bring some flexibility to the way K.M.'s system synchronized accommodation and convergence. K.M. was reevaluated a year later, in June 1981. The results showed that his vision system's ability in the areas worked on had improved greatly. As a consequence, the ability of his two eyes to work together as a team had also improved. K.M. happily reported that he did not have blurring or doubling when he read, the words stayed still and he didn't lose his place. The school district had reevaluated him and he was back in the general stream, after having spent a second summer at the school for the learning disabled. He was still being tutored in spelling and English.

Dr. Bazin was able to give K.M. a progress check in January 1984. He was still wearing the lenses for close work. His progress had continued. This was a confident K.M. who talked about the sports in which he was involved. His transition to junior high school had been successful. Not surprisingly, K.M.'s family was grateful for the therapy the youngster had received and told Dr. Bazin it was "the key that changed the course of his future." In conclusion, Dr. Bazin wrote:

As a new optometrist and more seasoned educator, I came to realize that the optometric intervention at that time made it possible for K.M. to respond to the educational remediation program.

This final point is an important one. Optometric vision therapy does not replace education, it does not "teach" youngsters how to read. Rather, it removes the obstacles that made it difficult or impossible for them to learn. Often, remedial education, tutoring, counseling or help such as occupational therapy will be needed after optometric vision therapy to help youngsters pull themselves into place.

Help For Dyslexics

The cause of dyslexia is not yet known. Research indicates a possible malfunction in the section of the brain responsible for sequencing. Because optometric vision therapy works with the neuromuscular, neurophysiological and neurosensory systems, this therapy is particularly valuable to youngsters and adults labeled dyslexic. Usually, dyslexics have problems like letter and word reversal. The letter *b* becomes a *p*, and *dad* turns into to *bad*. Or they may skip letters or parts of words, reading or writing *as* for *was*. These and other confusing errors make it practically impossible for dyslexics to function and achieve in the normal classroom setting or to be confident and have decent self-images.

Transforming An Eight-Year-Old Dyslexic

In his book *Total Vision*, Dr. Kavner discusses the case of a dyslexic boy who came to him for optometric vision therapy. The youngster was reading at first-grade level, two years behind his age group. He confused *b* with *d*, *no* for *on* and *saw* for *was* when reading and had no better luck with writing. A sensitive, lovable boy, he was disorganized to the point where he could not concentrate long enough to tie a shoelace. He often wandered around and would forget what he was supposed to be doing. Naturally, this caused parents and school a great deal of frustration, and it certainly didn't add to the boy's self-esteem. His sports ability was poor.

The visual exam showed that this youngster's eyes "actually lost the target when an object shifted from the left side of his body to the right. He lost visual contact with it until the other eye could locate it. Consequently, the two sides of his body were not cooperating smoothly, but always seemed as if one were fighting with the other." As so often happens with youngsters whose undiagnosed vision imbalances come to light through an optometric vision exam, once the boy was told he had a specific problem and that Dr. Kavner offered a way to treat it, he felt relieved and less frustrated and insecure. A daily program was organized which consisted of a series of "games" or exercises aimed at developing the coordination of both sides of his body with his eyes and developing his eyes' ability to guide body coordination. Office visits were scheduled for every two weeks.

By his second office visit, improvement was visible. The boy was happier and more outgoing. By the third and fourth sessions he was reporting enthusiastically on his newly found sports ability. Then, after four months, his reading ability suddenly leaped up to grade level (two grades). His ability for other subjects put him near the top of his classes. Dyslexia was no longer in the picture.

Total visits to the doctor's office: eight.

Total time elapsed: four months.

Dr. Kavner is the first to point out that such quick results do not happen all the time. Just sometimes.

Diagnosing Dyslexia

Behavioral optometrists were intrigued to read in the media on September 20, 1986, that an "eye movement test on pre-schoolers could provide a new tool for early diagnosis of dyslexia." They couldn't have agreed more. A professor of psychiatry and pediatrics at Rutgers University Medical School, Dr. George Pavlidis, presented the findings at a symposium on dyslexia held at The Gow School, America's oldest college preparatory school for dyslexic boys.

A report in the October 1, 1986 journal, *Education of the Handicapped*, said that dyslexia can be diagnosed in "preschool children through a computerized testing process that should be available commercially within a year. The technique uses a computer to trace, record and analyze eye movement patterns.... A two-year study conducted on both normal readers and severe dyslexics revealed irregular eye movement that differs significantly and consistently from normal readers."

The end product of the study is a computer program that tests, then gives the main strengths and weaknesses of the child, followed by a brief summary and recommendations. The study was hailed by David Gow, headmaster of the sixty-year-old Gow School, because it will help to identify dyslexic youngsters early. "Most of our kids come here in ninth or tenth grade. That's too late to start training people to read phonetically, the method used for teaching dyslexics to read," said the headmaster. Also, a "child will be spared the psychological problems and aversion to schooling" which often accompanies dyslexia. Important points but it is helpful to compare the differences between what this program and what optometric vision therapy have to offer for dyslexia.

Computer Program by Dr. Pavlidis
1. Tests eye movements.
2. Makes recommendations.

Optometric Vision Therapy
1. Tests entire vision system.
2. Makes recommendations.
3. Uses lenses & prisms.
4. Works with neuromuscular, neurophysiological and neurosensory systems to treat the causes of the dyslexia.

Starting On The Right Side When Writing English?

Mary was two months short of her sixth birthday when she was referred to behavioral optometrist Dr. Samuel Berne of Pennsylvania (now New Mexico). Her mother told Dr. Berne that her daughter was hyperactive and complained of headaches. Mary tilted her head when trying to read, had poor general coordination and the pupils of her eyes were large in normal light. The child reversed letters and numbers, was below average in copying skills and preferred to start from the right side when writing or copying.

Both the pediatrician and a neurologist had diagnosed Mary as having an attention deficit disorder, and Ritalin had been prescribed to control hyperactivity. When Dr. Berne discussed the situation with Mary's mother, she told him that she and her husband wanted a normal child, not a hyperactive one who needed to be controlled by Ritalin. The parents also hoped to place the child in a good private school. They feared that in her present condition, the youngster would not "fit" into a normal classroom environment.

Dr. Berne's visual examination showed that Mary had good visual acuity, 20/20, but that her eye movement was poor and she found it difficult to hold her focus. Her considerable head and body movement were attempts to compensate for poor visual abilities. Mary's eyes tended to break apart easily, unable to team or work together comfortable at close work. Now and then, she suppressed the use of one eye. After the exam, Dr. Berne was able to tell Mary's mother that the prognosis was good for her daughter's visual motor integration dysfunction to be treated with the correct lens use and also with in-office vision therapy. The parents and Dr. Berne agreed that:

1. Mary needed to learn to focus on the task at hand; much of her hyperactivity stemmed from her vision problems.

2. The family wished to reduce, then stop, the use of Ritalin.

3. Help was needed for Mary to learn to excel in a normal classroom environment.

Mary's Therapy Program

In the eight months that the youngster came to Dr. Berne's office for treatment, the program consisted of a variety of motor activities to help Mary develop the ability to focus on specific tasks. Together, Dr. Berne, his staff and Mary worked on chalkboard tracing and balancing on a 2 x 4 while focusing on a ball--all to the measured beat of a metronome. The aim was to develop an integration of both sides of the body through movement.

As Mary progressed with the therapy, she literally learned to "slow down." In one month, the child's hyperactivity had decreased by a good 60 percent and the parents were able to stop the use of Ritalin completely. Shortly thereafter, Mary's hyperactivity was completely eliminated. Once that stage was reached, Dr. Berne then worked on helping the youngster develop fine motor control in the areas of visual tracking, focusing, eye teaming and hand-eye coordination. Finally, the therapy covered visual thinking, imagery, and visualization.

A Home Program, Also

Dr. Berne prescribed lenses that incorporated a prism to improve Mary's ability to see detail. He also gave the youngster pinhole occluders (patches with a pinhole in) to be worn for one hour each day. Several other home procedures such as visual tracking were also used. Dr. Berne counseled the parents on the importance of setting limits for the child and also discussed how food allergies and sugar consumption can affect behavior. At the start of the school year, Mary was accepted by a Friends school and adjusted well to the classroom environment. She is no longer hyperactive and does not need to use Ritalin. The parents plan to visit Dr. Berne so that progress can be checked and also the lens prescription evaluated regularly to determine whether Mary's needs change.

Poor Handwriting, Poor Schoolwork, Poor Self-Esteem

Margaret, fifteen, went to Dr. Tirsa Quinones of Connecticut, for a behavioral vision evaluation in September 1985. A seventh grader, the youngster was having difficulties organizing her work and writing legibly. Margaret often had blurry vision and held reading material very to her eyes. Nonetheless, she enjoyed reading, which she did a lot. Throughout her school career, Margaret had had eye-hand coordination difficulties. The youngster had been wearing contact lenses for quite a while and also had single vision glasses. The exam revealed nearsightedness and even with the lenses prescribed before coming to Dr. Quinones, the youngster's visual acuity was slightly below the expected level, both at near and far distances. Margaret had difficulty changing focus from far to near, and focusing flexibility deteriorated when she read for long periods.

Margaret's two-eye depth perception and ability to use her eyes as a team for close work needed improvement. She also tended to overconverge her eyes at near--in other words, Margaret believed objects were closer to her than they really were. Her central and peripheral vision were not working as an integrated whole. As a consequence, Margaret tended to ignore peripheral information in order to complete nearpoint work. Tests showed poor use of central vision, as well as a significant suppression of visual information.

Dr. Quinones changed Margaret's spectacles to bifocals and also prescribed stress-relieving lenses to wear over her contact lenses while close work was being done. This brought increased visual acuity and improved some aspects of Margaret's visual performance, since she was not compensating so much for her nearsightedness. A less powerful prescription for close work was helpful. Optometric visual therapy was also recommended.

Peripheral Vision Is Essential

During the first sessions of the therapy, it was noted that while following, or tracking a slow moving target, the youngster would completely lose the object and look away--yet she was not aware that she had looked away. Margaret found it very difficult to be aware of peripheral information while attending to a task that needed the use of her central vision.

Awareness of the periphery is vital not only for basic survival reasons (Margaret, for instance, is a horse rider) but also for relieving the stress of sustained nearpoint work such as reading. People who observed Margaret horseback riding noted that she had little awareness of where she was in the ring and that she worked far harder than the norm to master the basic skills necessary in her sport. In the early therapy sessions, the youngster had to shift her feet on the balance board activities if she wanted to tip the board to the right, left, up or down positions, rather than shifting her weight off the central axis of her body. When using yoke prisms which provoked a perceptual shift of the environment up, down, right or left, she was unable to decode the large spatial changes caused by these prisms.

Margaret could not verbalize what she saw, and she did not show appropriate motor responses. She was confused, disoriented and made dizzy by these shifts. This suggested to therapist Joann Falbo that she was unable to decode and orient herself visually to changing spatial situations.

The youngster was unable to hold or fix her eyes in space accurately; her eyes drifted off target and she was not able to use sensory feedback to get back on target. When she made an error in visual problem solving, she would continue to repeat the error, unable to do something different. At such times, her frustration would be very intense.

During tachistoscopic tracings of forms (pictures exposed on a chalkboard for 1/10th, 1/50th or 1/100ths of a second), Margaret was asked to reproduce what she saw, where she saw it and how big she saw it. The task made her very anxious, and she would become confused by shapes and have difficulty in being accurate. Gradually, as the therapy progressed, Margaret began to develop appropriate visual motor responses and see and describe visual changes. By the end of approximately twelve months of therapy, Margaret had made the following changes:

- Visual acuity had improved to 20/20 both at far and near (with her lenses); near-sightedness had been reduced slightly and focusing flexibility was changed but was not fully satisfactory

- Two-eyed depth perception at near had gone from 60 percent to 100 percent

- Eye tracking full and smooth

- Had learned to direct herself accurately with her visual system and her spatial performance had become efficient; no longer misinterpreted location of objects

- No longer suppressed visual information and focusing ability as well as eye teaming showed wide ranges of flexibility and easiness

- Now understood mismatches and could use feedback and direct her actions in a more productive way

- Use of therapy lenses no longer uncomfortable

Home Therapy and Periodic Check-ups

At the end of the therapy program, Dr. Quinones outlined a maintenance program of activities for Margaret to continue at home and suggested that she come to the office for progress checks. Margaret's parents were happy to inform Dr. Quinones that the youngster's academic performance had improved. "Really doing well," was the comment. Just as important was the fact that Margaret was much happier with herself, her family and friends. Yet a few months earlier, she had tried to run away from home. One of the most significant changes was a reduction in the intensity with which she pursued a task. The frustration and anxiety she had shown in the past had diminished. In fact, Margaret had learned to deal with her work and her life in a relaxed, less stressful way because of the smoothness and balance in her vision system.

Underachievers

This is the case history of Amber Bennett. The youngster was having difficulty coping with her fourth-grade school work and had joined the ranks of school children described as under-achievers. In the summer after she finished fourth grade, Amber, who lived in Connecticut, went to the Gesell Institute for a vision analysis. By now, she'd had several routine eye examinations and had also been examined by one of the leading ophthalmologists in the area. No one had uncovered Amber's vision imbalances until she went to Gesell because until then the youngster had not been examined by anyone trained to evaluate the entire vision system and offer remedial therapy.

Mr. and Mrs. Bennett have four children. Their second youngest, Amber, is a happy affectionate girl. As a youngster, she was bubbly, cheerful and playful with her sisters, parents and friends. The first hint of any problem came when the youngster was tested for kindergarten at the age of five.

"You'll always have trouble with this child in school," the teacher informed Mrs. Bennett after the test. Astonished, Amber's mother asked why.

"She threw the pencil across the room."

Mrs. Bennett didn't mention the puzzling comment to her husband, although the words stayed in her mind for the next few days. Amber was such a happy child that soon the nagging thought was forgotten. Six years later, after Amber started optometric vision therapy, Mrs. Bennett realized that Amber was a youngster who had never settled down to crayoning or working with a pencil, connecting dots to dots, a favorite activity with her sisters. And Amber would wriggle off the lap of anyone who tried to read to her. Despite the warning comment from the teacher who'd given Amber the entrance test, Mrs. Bennett was relieved when Amber's year in kindergarten went smoothly. First grade was also pleasantly peaceful. A gradual change came in second grade. The teacher started to note problems. "Could do better. Work is good for five minutes then she talks and disrupts others."

By the end of second grade, school had given Amber a label. Her teacher liked the child but wrote that she was "lazy." Amber was also called "uncooperative." In third grade, the label changed. Amber was now identified as a "problem student." The teachers hastened to add that they liked her and the other children also got on well with Amber. It was just that she could not or would not concentrate on her work for more than a few minutes at a time. When she did work, the results were all right. But how can you finish anything when you keep stopping and chatting with friends?

During the routine eye test at school, when Amber was in fourth grade, the nurse suggested Amber might have trouble with her eyes. The school test used only the Snellen eye chart.

"Take the child for a thorough eye test," the nurse recommended. Mrs. Bennett asked friends for references and finally took Amber to the leading ophthalmologist in Fairfield county.

"Amber needs glasses. She has astigmatism but it's not really a problem," Mrs. Bennett was told. Amber wore the glasses for the rest of fourth grade. However, there was little change in the way she handled her schoolwork. That summer, a friend told Mrs. Bennett about the clinic at the Gesell Institute in New Haven that offered developmental, visual and physical evaluations for children aged 3 to 12. The institute, which was founded in 1911, had been operating a clinic since 1950. Mrs. Bennett had no hesitation in taking her daughter to Gesell for she had heard of its excellent reputation. This was just as well because the results of Amber's exam were shocking.

"Your child has several vision imbalances."

"Are you certain?" Mrs. Bennett said. "She was examined about six months ago and I was told her slight astigmatism wasn't a problem." Patiently, the optometrist who had examined Amber explained the situation.

Optometric Visual Analysis of Amber Bennett

Reverses and skips words.
Low attention span and difficulty concentrating in school.
Schoolwork below level.
Eyes reddened.

1. Difficulty in sustaining the two eyes converged; compensates by using excess effort and energy which results in a tendency for crossed eyes. [Only detectable by these tests, not visible to the naked eye.]

2. When looking in the distance, has difficulty in coordinating the two eyes. The left eye slips outwards when attempting to zero in on fine details. Extra effort must be used to pull the eyes together to avoid seeing double. When the left eye slips out, the vision in that eye is suppressed, otherwise she would be seeing double. Because of the disruption in the motor movement of the eyes, it is difficult for Amber to sustain focusing at close work for any length of time. Her focusing is spastic. This causes disruption in the child's ability to concentrate. These centers have a profound effect on the body's total motor system.

3. The disruption in visual performance described above results in classroom problems as well as general physical problems such as poor sleeping patterns, frequent indigestion and hyperactivity. Close work takes Amber a great deal of energy and effort and leads to rapid fatigue.

In October, Mrs. Bennett started taking Amber to Dr. Forkiotis once a week because his office was close to their home. At home, mother and daughter worked daily on specially prepared visual procedures.

"It was chaos," remembers Mrs. B. "I've always enjoyed running my home and bringing up four children. This was a totally different aspect of family life. At first, we didn't see results because there just weren't any. Changes were occurring, of course. But it was difficult to notice them. It was hard on Amber. She'd been seeing one way all her life and she'd been told that the procedures were to help change the way she saw. What could that mean to a fourth grader?

"Then, in February, we began to notice behavior changes. Also, Amber herself got very excited. Doctor Forkiotis told us one eye was starting to align. The result was an immediate improvement in Amber's memory retention of what she saw or read. We had our weekly visit. Doctor Forkiotis was very pleased with the progress so we were pleased, too. On the way home, I asked Amber a question, 'What is the difference between the eye the doctor says has aligned and the other one?' Without any hesitation, Amber replied, 'One eye doesn't have sides any more.'"

Mrs. Bennett laughs at the memory.

"I understood immediately what Amber meant," the mother recalls. "This was what Doctor Forkiotis had discussed with me. Up till now, my ten-year-old daughter had had 'tunnel' vision. She could hardly see out of the side of her eye. Her peripheral vision was very, very limited."

Within a few months, Amber's other eye had also responded to vision therapy. Eventually, the other symptoms of the youngster's visual problems were also corrected. Amber's behavior in the classroom changed. Her concentration expanded dramatically. Now, she was labeled a "good student," not a "troublemaker." The youngster was able to handle her schoolwork. Bad work habits also began to disappear, replaced by good ones.

How Long Does Therapy Usually Take?

Amber's visual imbalances were unusually serious, despite

her youth. Some youngsters with vision imbalances can be helped just by prescription of correct lenses to help reduce stress on the vision system or to support the system while it is developing. Others may benefit from a short course of vision therapy, some may need extended care. It all depends on the individual, the vision imbalances and the situation at home.

Dr. Apell says, "We have our failures as well as our successes. We will never be able to resolve all the problems that are brought to us. When there are other pressures on an individual in addition to vision imbalances, those pressures have to be dealt with for benefits to come from optometric vision therapy."

Underachievers come in different shapes and sizes. Those who struggle through school go on to greater struggles as adults. Maria, who had moved from New York to Oregon, went to Dr. Robert Pepper for optometric vision therapy. She had a painfully long list of troubles, which included alcoholism, a divorce, problems with her children and the loss of several jobs. She had sought a wide variety of professional help, including counseling, but everything had been of minimal help. At first, because of her vision imbalances, she had difficulty with the therapy. Dr. Pepper made tape recordings of each session .

"I'd call up Doctor Pepper in frustration to discuss why I was having difficulty with the home procedures. He'd ask if I had listened carefully to the instructions on the tape.

"Then, when I'd play back the tape, I'd find all the information there," said Maria. "I began to see why I'd had difficulties in the past."

Once the therapy was completed, Maria was astonished to find that her reactions to and perceptions of her family's behavior were very different.

"My vision imbalances had affected the way I perceived what went on around me. I had tried everything else but I still had major problems. Once we changed my vision system, the going was easier, in fact it was completely different."

20/20 Sight But A Poor Reader

Many individuals do not have obvious problems such as blurred sight, or headaches, yet often an examination of the complete system reveals vision imbalances. Some people are motivated and succeed despite problems, although inevitably they will pay a high price. They may be tense or perpetually anxious, perhaps they will ultimately need tranquilizers. Others may turn to drug use or abuse or alcohol dependency; for some it may be the common garden variety of irritability or inability to be on good terms with the world. Some may be cheerful types but chronically unable to cope. They may be habitually late, or forgetful, or unable to keep up with the demands of their routine. Vision imbalances exert their toll eventually in myriad subtle ways.

A profile on someone who had no complaints about vision problems was in the March 1984 *Optometry Times* column, "My Most Interesting Case," by Martin Birnbaum, O.D., Associate Professor at the State University of New York College of Optometry and a noted writer and lecturer in the field.

Chris, a seventeen-year-old boy with a history of reading problems since first grade, was seen for a routine optometric examination. He did not have any complaints and had no difficulty reading the chalkboard or small print. Despite extensive tutoring, he had major problems in reading, especially in comprehension. At the beginning of the optometric exam, the first results were normal. By the end of the complete analysis of the entire vision system, significant inadequacies were revealed in accommodative and binocular fusion. In the case history of K.M, by Dr. Bazin earlier in this chapter, these problems caused blurring, double vision and difficulty in keeping the right place when reading. Chris did not exhibit any of these symptoms although his vision system had inadequacies similar to K.M. Chris also had an intermittent suppression of the left eye. Dr. Birnbaum found that the visual perceptual motor testing showed expected levels. Chris was six years below the level expected for his age on an oral reading test. He left out or made mistakes on small words. He disliked reading and did as little of it as possible.

The vision therapy was designed to work on the specific problems. Chris came in for office visits but also worked on home procedures which consolidated the progress made under the optometrist's care. Lenses were prescribed for close work such as reading. Chris responded rapidly and was able to stop treatment after three months. He developed a greater interest in reading and found it easier to do for long periods without difficulty. His reading skills showed major improvements. Chris decided to go to college, something he had not previously considered. Dr. Birnbaum's conclusion stresses an important point that applies to many.

Small word errors and omissions are quite common among patients with functional vision disorders at near-point. These problems may reflect a tendency to scan globally rather than to focus on detail when reading.... Cases such as this one are extremely common and treatment is simple and straightforward. Success rates are extremely high. Why, then, do I cite Chris as one of my most interesting cases?

This case stresses the fallacy of treating or referring for vision therapy only those patients who report...symptoms. Many patients read little and poorly as a result of their vision problems, yet they experience few symptoms because they read so little. Complete optometric evaluation, including assessment of accommodative and binocular function, must be performed on all patients, not merely on those with...complaints.

To do less is to deny care that has a significant capacity to expand human potential.

Chapter 6

Eyes On Camelot

They called it Camelot. The revival of a magic realm in the twentieth century, a democratic kingdom whose rulers were rich and powerful. Their influence spread from Washington throughout the land and across the seas to foreign lands. Yet there was trouble in the palace. Terrible trials had befallen the family of the king's first aide, one of the most powerful men in Washington.

One of the family's beloved daughters appeared to be under a spell, to be cursed so that nothing she did went well. She could not read. She could not study. She could not learn. Happiness and peace of mind seemed beyond her reach. In their despair, the family had turned first here, then there. They had called upon physicians, psychiatrists, ophthalmologists, educators--to no avail. At last, a wise and learned woman, physician to the King, came forth to counsel the family.

In the beginning, the family thought her advice was in vain.

"We have tried that cure," the mother and father said, sadly.

"No," replied the physician. "You did not consult the correct person."

And behold! This was sage advice. When the beloved daughter went to the correct person, troubles were found that were hidden from the other sages. He saw that the daughter had sight but not vision. Where the other sages had pronounced that sight was enough, this practitioner knew differently. He employed his battery of skills upon the daughter. And lo! A change came over her. She could read. She could concentrate. She could learn. Her life brightened and rounded. Her family gave thanks.

The beloved daughter was Luci Baines Johnson. When she was a teenager and her father vice president of the United States, Luci was having serious problems with her schoolwork. Her parents, classic overachievers, were deeply worried. Despite their wealth, despite their access to all kinds of learned advice, despite having explored every possible avenue, nothing they tried had helped. Tutoring, remedial education, counseling, they had tried everything. It had reached the point where Luci became nauseous when she had to sit and try to do her homework. On academic probation, with a foreign language exam coming up that she had to pass, Luci worked with a tutor. Her score was perfect, because she worked hard, as she always did--but also because the tutor did not use written material; everything was auditory. At the end of the days of tutoring, Luci was told, "You could not have failed this subject before, you are one of the best students I've ever had."

"Please tell my parents that," came the reply.

The tutor did, and the parents revived the question again. How could Luci be helped? What was the problem? Then Janet Travell, M.D., President Kennedy's personal physician, suggested that Luci's vision might be at the center of the maze. Luci's parents responded that her eyes had been checked and she had 20/20 sight. Dr. Travell pointed out that Luci's vision had not been analyzed. As a result, Luci was sent to a

Washington optometrist who specialized in optometric vision therapy. A small miracle happened from Luci's point of view. Once she had completed a program of the therapy she went from academic probation to honor roll. It took time, of course, and work. She recalls that she could not at first understand what the various procedures had to do with her schoolwork. She trained with such aids as stereoptic machines and a ticking metronome for rhythmic eye movements.

"If my family, with its wealth and power, could seek so long and unsuccessfully for the right answer to my problem, how many others throughout our country also seek this help?" asked Luci Baines Johnson. In her gratitude, this young woman then gave her time as a volunteer for several summers in the office of Dr. Robert Kraskin, the optometrist who had helped her. Luci also has spoken to audiences about the value of optometric vision therapy.

"If the key to a better society is education, the key to a better education is better vision. If you don't have that key, you can't open the door to a better life."

Who Are the Practitioners?

Once you identify, or even suspect, the presence of a vision problem, who do you turn to for help?

Two kinds of practitioners offer eye care:

- An *optometrist* whose doctoral degree is O.D., doctor of optometry

- An *ophthalmologist* whose doctoral degree is M.D., doctor of medicine (and who specializes in diseases of the eye and surgery)

The O.D. degree is earned after a minimum of seven years of college and graduate education. Optometric education begins with a preoptometry program which is almost identical to premed and predental programs, with the exception of the more stringent requirements in mathematics and psychology for the

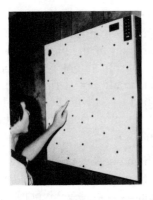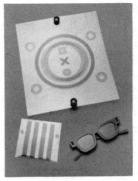

Equipment for optometric vision therapy can be as simple as a ball on a string or as technical as the Wayne Computerized Saccadic Fixator on the left or the binocularity kit on the right.

optometry student. A comparison is made in Appendix I of typical professional programs in optometry, dentistry and medicine. Optometry's areas of specialization range from contact lenses to pediatric vision. Perhaps one of the most innovative is that of behavioral optometry, for which postdoctoral training is needed.

- General optometrists offer routine eye health care and refraction (the clinical measurement of the eye to determine the need for lenses).

Their extensive education has prepared general optometrists to detect not only ocular diseases but signs of certain health problems such as hypertension, diabetes and arteriosclerosis. The location of optometrists in communities of all types and sizes offers the public an invaluable primary health care which is conveniently accessible.

- Behavioral optometrists (including functional or developmental) practice optometric vision therapy, sometimes in addition to general optometry, sometimes exclusively.

In contrast to general optometrists and ophthalmologists, who usually believe that visual problems stem from random or genetic biological variations, behavioralists believe that visual problems may be triggered by environmental factors that include developmental or stress-induced factors as well as genetic factors.

While the basic concepts of behavioral, functional and developmental optometry are essentially the same, there are certain differences in the therapeutic approaches. Dr. Martin Birnbaum wrote in the *Journal of Optometric Vision Development* in March 1986, in his article, "Perspectives on Behavioral Optometry," "while the functionalist tends to view vision disorders in terms of ocular and oculomotor function...the behavioral optometrist views vision disorders as more holistically interrelated with general behavior... the behavioral optometrist is aware of relationships between vision and movement, balance, posture, orientation and localization in space, spatial judgments, and perception."

In broad terms, all optometrists analyze eye health and refractive conditions. The type of prescriptions they write for lenses (glasses or contacts) varies and depends on the concepts in which they believe. By the fall of 1990, all fifty states in America had licensed optometrists to use diagnostic pharmaceuticals and twenty-five states had expanded this to include treatment of eye conditions with therapeutic pharmaceuticals.

Ophthalmologists are medical doctors who specialize in diseases of the eye; most also practice eye surgery. Ophthalmologists, like optometrists, also examine eyes and prescribe lenses. Their training, however, is in treating diseases of the eye primarily with drugs and surgery although orthoptics is part of the ophthalmologic regimen.

To recap, here are definitions:

Optometrist —A doctor of optometry (O.D.) educated to provide routine eye health care and refraction.

Behavioral Optometrist—A doctor of optometry (O.D.) whose postdoctoral training is in optometric vision therapy, which involves a wide variety of procedures for neuromuscular, neurophysiological, or neurosensory visual dysfunction.

Ophthalmologist—A doctor of medicine (M.D.) whose postdoctoral training is in diseases of the eye and surgery.

Optician— A technician who produces and/or dispenses the optical lenses, glasses or other equipment prescribed by optometrists and ophthalmologists.

Who Needs Which Practitioner?

"Routine eye care is required by everyone. It involves infrequent visits which are predictable," wrote Dr. Nathan Flax in "Vision Therapy and Insurance: A Position Statement," published by the State College of Optometry in New York in 1986. "Vision therapy, on the other hand, is not required by all people. It often involves extended care to treat a diagnosed...condition." An optometrist will routinely refer you to an ophthalmologist if eye disease is discovered or suspected. You will need the care of an ophthalmologist for surgery, of course, but general eye care is well taken care of by general optometrists. If you have any of the symptoms of vision problems discussed in this book, the practitioner of choice is the optometrist who offers vision therapy.

How Does Optometric Vision Therapy Work?

This drug-free therapy is effective because it treats the cause of the problem not merely the symptom. When Dr. Edelman prescribes help for migraine sufferers, he is not working with the symptoms, the migraine, he works with the area that is causing the symptom. When Dr. Forkiotis prescribes help for a youngster having trouble learning, he is not offering educational help, he works with the area causing the blockage to learning. When any practitioner of optometric vision therapy treats any individual with a vision imbalance, the help is for the cause of the problem. This is a preventive health therapy, just as dentistry is preventive health care.

Optometric vision therapy works with the vision system and the various subsystems that integrate with vision. The vision system, for which the eyes are the external receptors, is the prime connection between the body's central control, the brain, and the activities going on around us. Eye-brain communication is possible because the retina is the only tissue in the entire body derived from the brain during the embryonic and fetal stages.

> *When your eyes are examined with a retinoscope by the optometrist who practices vision therapy, it is quite literally an examination of the way your brain functions. Ultimately, the vision system creates the eye-brain-behavior connection. When optometrists treat you with vision therapy, they are in effect working with the brain, the body's central control.*

William M. Ludlam, O.D., an optometrist from Hillsboro, Oregon, discusses the mechanics of how optometric vision therapy works with the brain in "Vision Therapy and Insurance." "Vision, the dominant sense of man, is dependent on coordinated eye movement for its proper functioning." Dr. Ludlam explained that three separate control systems, individually located in different places in the brain, are each responsible for the control of a separate eye muscle system's movement.

"Each of these three systems may have defects, either individually or as a group and the development of proper coordination and control of these three... functions is a major aim of optometric vision therapy." Dr. Ludlam was not presenting a new concept. Far from it. Others before him, both in behavioral optometry and in medicine, had outlined the thesis that vision is a process that takes place at the brain level. Of course, the behavioral optometrists are unique in their development of an effective therapy.

The Mental Process Of Seeing

A. D. Ruedemann, M.D., Chairman of the Department of Ophthalmology at Wayne State University College of Medicine, presented the Chairman's Address at an American Medical Association meeting in June 1956. Among other things, Dr. Ruedemann said: "The fovea [point in the retina where vision is most acute] is the center of sight for stimulating the learning process. Following this there must be visual memory and fusion. The entire system forms a nucleus for most of our intelligence and thought process."

Dr. Ruedemann also noted that vision and learning are integral to each other, and the vision system is a whole that must be treated in a certain way. He stated his opposition to surgery for vision imbalances in no uncertain terms:

> *It has been nearly two centuries since that charlatan Taylor started us off on the wrong foot, or perhaps the wrong eye, by cutting eye muscles.... This has been a serious handicap because it has led people away from the basic physiology in the mental process of seeing.*

> *The fact of the matter is that seeing is a learning process. No one is born knowing how to see.*

Learning To See

The concept that vision is a process that can be developed is basic to behavioral optometry. Optometric vision therapy helps the vision system learn to work in the most balanced way possible. You might compare it with taking math lessons or learning to play sports. We accept the need to learn academic subjects or sports. The same is true of vision. Yes, we can see but we must learn to use our vision systems so that we understand what we see.

Dr. Ruedemann pointed out that it is the rare individual who benefits from surgery to correct vision imbalances. Surgery has its place, in particular where there is muscle paralysis (this affects less than 2 percent of the population in the United States). If it is considered appropriate for cosmetic purposes, be aware that all too often the surgery causes temporary change. This is because the cause has not been treated, only the symptom. The brain soon makes an adjustment to the new muscle lengths created by the surgery and the eye usually moves to a new position, still not in balance with the other eye.

In situations where learning, behavior and health difficulties have not responded to other therapies, it is wise to seek the counsel of an optometrist who practices vision therapy. Even more preferable, practice preventive care and consult behavioral optometry before problems arise, since this practice offers the most comprehensive examination of the vision system and has effective, noninvasive therapy.

Our Two-Way Link: The Eye

In his book, *Vision: Its Development in Infant and Child,* Arnold Gesell, M.D., wrote: "... the eye is...the most direct corridor to the vast networks of the brain cortex, where billions of neurons organize and engender the energies which issue in vision. Inconceivably intricate electronic events take place when this amazing complex of structures is stirred into reaction."

The American Optometric Association joins the Gesell Institute and other organizations such as the Optometric Extension Program Foundation in reiterating that vision is learned. The ability to see and correctly interpret what is seen does not appear automatically at birth. It develops over a lifetime and is shaped by your experiences and environment.

The Analysis Of The Vision System

On your first visit, you will complete a personal history form. This will include information on motor development, general health, and details on education as well as social and emotional development. Then comes the analysis of the vision system. The initial departure from the norm comes with the interpretation of the retinoscope exam, in which differences in visual responses are detected. The range includes:

- Dullness and brightness of the reflex

- Reflex color (from dull red to white)

- Speed, range, promptness, pick-up and release of motion

The behavioral optometrist makes a series of other tests in addition to the retinoscope exam. This is described as "probing" the system. Usually, a minimum of twenty-one aspects of the vision system and the way it works are analyzed, as well as the accommodative process (the way the lens changes focus), the convergence process, and the way these two mechanisms work together and interact. It is particularly important to form a picture of the quality of the system's activity. This is done by comparing reactions to a norm. Values above or below the normal limits may show a pattern or syndrome.

Lenses and prisms are used during the vision analysis. Lenses have a specific effect on the accommodative pattern, while prisms expand or compress the perceptual view and thus change behavior. Tests are made to evaluate how your vision system handles the visual process. These include book retinoscopy, bell retinoscopy, objective as well as subjective measurements of oculomotor control, evaluation of accommodative facility and a series of stereoscopic measurements of the quality of how well your two eyes fuse input. Other evaluations analyze strabismus or amblyopia. A final phase covers measurements of central processing skills: spatial orientation, visual discriminations and interpretations, intersensory motor matching, visual recall and visualization.

The results help determine what type of care is necessary. Perhaps you will need lenses (glasses or contacts), or you might need to go to the office for therapy. A combination of lenses and therapy is also a possibility.

Different Concepts, Different Prescriptions

The lenses prescribed for optometric vision therapy are quite different from those used by the general optometrist or the ophthalmologist. In general, the latter two groups use lenses in one way only. They prescribe compensating lenses. For instance, if a child is nearsighted (commonly a symptom of a vision imbalance), compensating lenses can provide 20/20 sight. But as the imbalance grows, as it almost always does, stronger and stronger lenses usually have to be prescribed to maintain 20/20 sight because the vision imbalance is still there. Since this approach is sight-oriented, the underlying causes of the nearsightedness (or whatever the symptom) are not being treated. The vision system is not being brought into balance, which might eliminate the need for these compensating lenses.

Preventive, Developmental or Remedial Lenses

Behavioral optometrists, in contrast, prescribe lenses in various ways:

- Preventive lenses to prevent a problem in the vision system from starting in those individuals diagnosed "at risk"

- Developmental lenses to support and nurture an immature vision system while helping it develop normally and cope with visual stress

- Remedial lenses for a specific situation (such as an inability to sustain focusing) until that ability is adequate

How Lenses Help

Lenses and prisms act by changing the value and quality of the light gradients as they enter the eye. Changes in input result in changes in output, depending on previously learned experience. The value of the lenses and prisms, therefore, is in their ability to alter to varying degrees the motor output of the organism. Lenses primarily alter the output responses of the somatic nervous system:

- Anti-stress lenses help fight the symptoms of stress.

- "Plus" lenses protect youngsters from developing vision imbalances.

A convex (curving outward) plus lens, applied in gradually increasing powers, causes dramatic results. When the acceptable lens power is reached, back tensions reduce, neck and head oscillations cease and other behaviors return to normal.

In *Optometry Times* of May 1985, Dr. Nathan Flax wrote that "in some cases, the use of a low-power lens to help attain accommodation at near point has been helpful in retarding the progression of myopia." Dr. Flax also explains that: "the amount of stress on the visual system from sustained close work is a product of time on the job, intensity of the demand, difficulty of the material, and the intellectual capacity of the individual. Under this stress, one response is a tendency for the patient to move the material closer. However, since the accommodative system receives its innervation from the parasympathetic branch of the autonomic nervous system--the branch that goes into decline during emotional arousal--focusing becomes more difficult. Therefore, although the individual wants to get closer to the material for the purpose of staying in rapport with the task, it becomes increasingly difficult to focus."

Now a cycle develops. As it becomes more difficult for you to focus, this affects your ability to converge your eyes, or turn them inward so you can see an object close to you. If, as a result of stress, you have difficulty focusing and you begin to strain to focus, you send signals of strain to the convergence system. You overconverge, and then have to adjust by bringing the head even closer. Now you need to focus differently. It's a wearying circle that doesn't take you anywhere. But it can make your vision system tense and eventually can become a permanent imbalance. This spills over into health and behavior, too.

A pioneer in the field of developmental lenses for children, Dr. Richard Apell has also written extensively on the subject. In a paper in *The Science Counselor* of September 1956, Dr. Apell explained that the traditional compensating lenses that "corrected" nearsightedness so that a child could see the chalkboard and other distant objects clearly actually overstimulated the focusing ability. Eventually, you ended up with an increase in the nearsightedness.

Dr. Apell explains that developmental lenses are always plus lenses. They have a very specific effect. When you look at something close to you, two different visual functions are involved: pointing, or centering, and focusing. The plus lens will allow you to point or center your vision at one distance while focusing at another. Usually, this is very comfortable for the vision system, although occasionally, some individuals will have different needs that can be met with a variation in the lens prescription.

Habit-forming Lenses?

This question is often asked. We are accustomed to the fact that traditional compensating lenses often become a necessity. However, developmental lenses are entirely different. The answer is, " No, you won't find developmental lenses habit-forming." You will find they are like good shoes or a baseball glove, comfortable and supportive. When youngsters who have worn such lenses have been examined after six to eight weeks, often improved visual performance is found.

When tested without their lenses, the youngsters have improved visual acuity, depth perception and convergence. They have also stopped complaining about being unable to read for more than ten minutes before the words blur. Their level of concentration has grown from a few minutes to a respectable period of time and headaches have disappeared, often completely. Their teachers and their families find them willing to cooperate and less tense.

Dr. Apell reminds us that developmental lenses are not a panacea for the myriad visual problems found among school-children. "A glove would not be of much use to the baseball player who did not know how to play baseball. The case is the same when the child lacks such basic visual skills as the ability to change focus rapidly from far to near, to fixate rapidly from far to near or from side to side, to maintain fixation on a moving target, or to coordinate the vision of the right eye with that of the left in all these activities. If youngsters cannot perform adequately in these basic areas of vision, we can hardly expect them to achieve easily the complex visual skills involved in securing meaning and understanding from printed symbols."

Individuals vary from situation to situation. The vision system is dynamic, ever moving, ever adjusting. In youngsters, the development of the system is an ongoing function. In adults, the daily routine has its effect on vision, but more importantly, the adult must live with any visual inadequacies present from childhood. Imbalances don't go away. You learn to accommodate to them, just as you would learn to accommodate a limp.

A Therapy Program

A carefully designed program tailored specifically to the individual can:

- Help prevent the development of some vision problems, such as myopia

- Aid in the proper development of vision abilities

- Enhance the efficiency and comfort of vision functioning

- Help correct existing vision problems

When To Have the First Exam?

Early in life, certainly no later than the age of four. If problems are suspected, it's never too early. Although no one is suggesting that infants be given glasses or contacts to wear, they can actually be helped by the behavioral optometrist, with external aids, right in the practitioner's office. Their systems are so young and plastic, they respond rapidly.

In general, it's good to have a youngster examined before the demands of school have begun. This gives the optometrist an opportunity to appraise the natural visual development up to that point and to make suggestions about the kinds of eye-hand activities that will encourage optimal visual development, these are included in Chapter 8. A second exam a year later will be compared to the first. This comparison reveals the direction and rate of visual development and provides an opportunity for additional suggestions about visual activities.

Once a child begins school, it's wise to consider protective lenses. Certain ages have crucial phases in the development of vision and when you add the demands of school, you have the potential for problems. Children may have one of several reactions in their vision. If they make demands of themselves, they may become nearsighted--they force their system to meet their demands. If such an adaptation is too painful, they may opt to withdraw from schoolwork and suddenly develop a dislike for school. The ages and stages of development are discussed in Chapter 8. The key point is that it's never too late to bring some balance to your vision, but like anything else, an early start saves grief.

Vision pervades a person's entire emotional and physical makeup and, as Dr. Hans Selye has shown, every part of the body tries to adapt to prolonged stress. Charles Cerami wrote in *Woman's Day* of April 1966, "A muscle that is loaded with increasing burdens strengthens in order to bear them; a person who spends long hours in the cold gets increased thyroid activity to produce more internal heat, and his skin learns to contract to cut heat loss. And all this is directed by a central intelligence center in the brain that receives information, analyzes it, and sends back commands. Can the [vision system] be any different, any less a part of the whole flexible system?"

Dr. Jean-Paul Blouin, a Canadian behavioral optometrist, summed up the results of visual problems:

When a person is handicapped in any visual task because of a visuomotor problem, or when fatigue is building up within his organism because of an excessive energy consumption related to visual work, his behavior tends to deteriorate. He becomes more nervous and more irritated. He may even lose his temper and become erratic in his behavior.

Who is affected by this problem? Not only the individual himself but his spouse, children, parents, brothers and sisters, teachers, classmates, playmates and workmates. Any or all of them may have to pay for the inconvenience of disturbed behavior.

The use of multifocal lenses can improve visuomotor development, increase resistance to fatigue and help one to become or to remain more sociable. This might be the whole difference between being a happy person or a nuisance to everybody.

Multifocal Lenses

The ideal lens for near and the one for far obviously are different. The lens for near work is stronger in positive power than the one for far. Thus, a multifocal lens offers a convenient, comfortable choice. Adults are often surprised that such a lens is suggested for youngsters, but when it has benefits for the individual, the choice is clear. Since such a multifocal lens is prescribed for developmental or anti-stress purposes, it is not likely that it will become a permanent part of the youngster's needs for it will eventually help strengthen certain visual abilities. Then the lenses can be discarded.

What Is Therapy Like?

As Mr. Cerami wrote, the diversity of procedures "stress the interplay of all the body's systems, and especially the hand and eye relationships. So an office where vision therapy is given seems, at first glance, more like a playroom than a clinic. One child teeters on a balance-board, while staring at a rotating multicolored disc. Two others play an ordinary game of checkers, but they are peering through eyeglasses with one red lens and one green. Still another looks into a machine that was first invented to teach our airmen how to recognize enemy planes in a flash; the boy tries to record six-digit numbers as they flit by at one one-hundredth of a second."

Perhaps this does not sound like a realistic task? Dr. Gesell wrote in 1949 that in baseball one fixes one's eyes yet also poises them for sudden unpredictable shifts. "The ball speeds across the plate in 3/10 of a second. The batter has 1/50 of a second in which to connect." Some four decades later, we've accelerated performance time. Roger Bannister's mile speed has been overtaken. By the same token, we've intensified our academic workload and streamlined our tools; the computer is chipping away at the pen's ubiquity. Optometric vision therapy has also expanded its repertoire of equipment.

Often, lenses or prisms are used while patients work on their tasks. Mark might use training lenses that create an extra image as he tries to see the letters on a ball that rotates in a circle at the end of a string. As he follows the ball's movement, he bobs and weaves and slowly the awkward movements acquire a dancer's grace. In time he will even learn to hold two long sticks a hairbreadth from the slowly moving ball. Sometimes, one piece of equipment can work on different imbalances. The translid binocular interactor is helpful in improving several problems, including diminished and low vision, eyes that turn in or out or do not point in the same direction when covered and vision suppression. Therapy equipment comes in a variety of shapes and sizes. The Bernell Corporation of Indiana filled the first thirty-three pages of its 1990 catalog with products for vision therapy.

In this therapy, lens and prism use are combined with a wide diversity of procedures. The tasks vary widely, depending on the individual's special needs. Some, such as walking on a balance beam or jumping on a trampoline, will seem like play. Others make use of equipment that is space age in its sophistication. Repetition of these tasks is aimed at improving vision by improving the interaction of all the sensory motor activities with vision at the helm. Some of the therapy may appear as simple as the physical movements of hip, shoulder and back muscles.

At the 1985 Northeast Vision Conference in Northampton, Massachusetts, Dr. Blouin outlined a visuomotor training program which he had found of benefit for patients with a variety of vision imbalances. His was not a new approach for optometric vision therapy, but his lecture was an original and stirring presentation of the material, in which he related the connection of the program to our progressive evolution and biological changes. Rolling, rocking, modified pushups, creeping, crawling and "crab" walking all have their place in bringing balance to the distortions imposed on us by vision dysfunction. It is this connection that makes somatic training such as Feldenkrais or shiatsu so valuable. Preventive health care interacts to enhance our abilities and performance.

Full-Spectrum Light, An Unsung Necessity

You won't put on weight with this nutrient and it's good for your health to have as much of it as possible. Researchers are finding that the correct type of light, specific wavelengths, is valuable to our health. Dr. Larry Wallace, a behavioral optometrist in Ithica, New York, explains why full-spectrum light is valuable for us. "Light is a major form of energy and nutrition just like air, food and water. It is necessary for optimal visual, physical, mental and emotional well being."

UPI Health Editor Patricia McCormack wrote in a series of dispatches published in 1981 that healthful light is full spectrum sunlight or the full-spectrum artificial light. She listed the problems documented in scientific studies that mal-illumination or insufficient equivalent sunlight or full-spectrum light can:

- Cause interference with calcium absorption (in animals and humans)

- Contribute to brittle bones in senior citizens

- Cause jaundice in newborns

- Increase tooth decay and rickets in youngsters

Too much of the wrong kind of artificial light can cause biorhythms to get out of step. This leads to:

- Problems with youngsters in school

- Reduced productivity in office and factory workers

So you were absolutely correct when you thought you felt off color in the dark days of winter. Small wonder the Russians have mandated use of full-spectrum light in many workplaces. In schools in Russia, it has been shown that full-spectrum lighting or ultraviolet treatment helps academic performance and student behavior and is accompanied by lower fatigue. The Russians also use light therapy on coal miners who spend their working day out of natural light. The treatment does more than prevent or treat black lung disease. It also helps the lungs clear themselves.

In West Germany, the government restricts use of cool, white low-spectrum light in public buildings because of its distorted spectral output.

Vision and Light

The impact of good or bad light on health is considerable. During the 1980s, we had more and more reports in the media, including the *New York Times*, on how scientists were discovering the value of full-spectrum light for individuals who've struggled with chronic depression. Where other therapies had failed, light was effective in dispelling the depression. One point consistently emerged, though. The amount of light and length of the treatment needed varied greatly from patient to patient. Perhaps one factor here is the efficiency of the patients' vision systems.

The optic nerve has two major pathways after it leaves the eye. One is a visual pathway transmitting photoelectric impulses to the brain's cortex, where vision perception and sight occur. The other is a nonvisual or energetic pathway that leads to the hypothalamus, pineal and pituitary glands. These glands regulate endocrine and autonomic function and therefore are responsible for physical and emotional changes. A small percentage of light is ultimately used to trigger the specific endocrine glands which cause physical and emotional changes--but even though it's a small percentage, if it's not full-spectrum light, you will be deprived of the value of light as a nutrient. Also, if your vision system has imbalances, light absorption will be affected.

What are the solutions? Do we all have to migrate to sunnier climes? Not necessarily. Behavioral optometry is careful to avoid most tinting in lens use because in general, tinting reduces the spectrum of light. Green lenses, for example, let through only green wavelengths and you are overdosing on green light and not receiving a balanced spectrum of all the other wavelengths. Pink is a tint to avoid. Scientific studies show related health problems (excessive calcium deposits in heart tissue, greater tumor development, and a strong tendency toward irritable and aggressive behavior) from the use of pink lenses or lights.

Optometrists who practice vision therapy will often suggest you try to spend a certain amount of time outside each day. An hour is good. This doesn't mean one has to be in direct sunlight; you can get the full benefit of natural daylight by sitting or reading under a shade tree or eating on a screened porch. Avoid too frequent use of sunglasses. Top-quality sunglasses are those with lenses which are full-spectrum neutral gray, manufactured by Keystone Optical Laboratory. If you find strong light painful, this may be an aspect of vision dysfunction. It's your body's way of signaling for help. Anti-stress lenses can bring a measure of relaxation to the system and often eliminate that discomfort.

Full-spectrum light bulbs or fluorescent tubes are available in a range of sizes to fit into your existing fixtures. Check local health food stores; they can often order them for you. Today's housing often has areas like kitchens and bathrooms with little natural light. In these cases, the use of full-pectrum lighting is an excellent idea. In 1985, the New York Association for the Blind reported favorably on Finnish lighting imports available from Pencar of Flushing, New York. They were of particular benefit for diabetics, who must be able to see a color match strip accurately. The value of full-spectrum lighting is that it gives vivid, true color with less glare. The *New York Times* reported in April 1986 that "Neodymium bulbs imported from Finland have a bluish, instead of clear glass envelope, which absorbs yellow tones put out by the filament, resulting in a cooler light source and excellent color reading. It also is a superb light for reading."

Another source of quality full-spectrum light fixtures is Environmental Systems of Lancaster, Pennsylvania. The fixtures are made to the design specifications of Dr. John Ott, a major figure in the field of full-spectrum light and its effect on health. Some of the fixtures are utilitarian in design but acceptable for basement, kitchen or bathroom. If your decor demands more style, the appearance of the fixtures' metal casings could be changed by painting or staining them or adding wood moldings.

John Ott spent the better part of four decades observing the effect light has upon plant growth. He was prompted to this type of research by his work with time-lapse photography for Walt Disney films. Dr. Ott's curiosity was aroused when he realized that the plants he was photographing were flourishing, despite the lack of natural light (he was working in a window-less basement). Ultimately, he created full-spectrum fluorescents by the addition of the correct amount of black light to the phosphors used in fluorescent tubes.

In September 1986, the *Reader's Digest* warned that recent "scientific investigation indicates there is a dark side to light, particularly the types of light used so widely in our schools, factories and offices." The *Digest* suggested that the "public should be informed of the potential hazards of artificial light." A final illuminating point, although the full-spectrum light bulbs or fixtures may be more expensive to buy than regular equipment, they are less expensive to operate and last longer. Best of all, full-spectrum light is a valuable, nonfattening nutrient.

No Quick Answers

At a 1985 seminar in California, one of the many held regularly throughout the world by the OEP Foundation, Dr. Getman summed up the main reason why behavioral optometry resists attempts made to explain the therapy in simple terms or efforts to treat people quickly.

"I've spent decades looking for the fast, easy way to offer optometric vision therapy. No quick answer exists. No shortcut is possible. No two people are exactly alike or have exactly the same set of problems."

Dr. Getman reminded his audience that each individual needs a careful, thorough optometric vision analysis. The length of time needed either for lenses or vision therapy will vary. Unless the individual has the motivation to wear the lenses or practice the procedures regularly, scant success can be expected. Dr. Streff once commented that not every individual is a candidate for optometric vision therapy. "Motivation is essential." If someone doesn't want to work to see better or is not able to understand they have a vision problem, no one can do the work for him or her. Other factors which influence the outcome of therapy are health, your family situation and your background. One young man who had dropped out of high school when he was fifteen had been very successful in starting his own business, a comic store. Then, he wrote, illustrated and published a comic book, which he expanded into a successful series. He then decided he would like to attend art school. Despite his obvious ability as an artist, his success in handling his business and the creation of a comic book series, lack of academic success counted against him. He was refused admission to the college of his choice. Up to that point, he had been content to live with nearsightedness. By chance, Colin Dawkins, the writer's husband, frequented the comicbook store. Colin and his friend John Severin, an internationally acknowledged artist, had collaborated on a series of comics. In fact, Colin had known and worked with many of the greats in the comic world for decades.

An enthusiastic and firm supporter of optometric vision therapy, Colin suggested that the young man give the therapy a chance. With the help of a behavioral optometrist, the young man worked hard to change the vision imbalance which was causing his nearsightedness. He was successful. This story doesn't end with the young man reapplying to college and being accepted. Instead, he turned to expanding his business and creating more comics. He is, in fact, comfortable being a success.

Help For Those With Physical Disabilities

Optometric vision therapy has brought substantial improvements for those inflicted with severe handicaps, from the visually impaired to those devastated by traumatic brain injury. These changes are exciting not only because they significantly improved the individuals' and their families' quality of life but because such changes had not been expected by the traditional health care practitioners. It was behavioral optometry that opened up the possibilities.

Dr. William V. Padula, an optometrist who directs the Low Vision Clinic of the Easter Seal Rehabilitation Center in New Haven, Connecticut, is also a consultant to programs serving disabled persons across the United States and in Mexico. He specializes in behavioral vision care for those with visual impairments, multihandicaps and traumatic brain injury. Dr. Padula is on the staff of the Woodmere Hospital for Traumatic Brain Injury in Connecticut and also has a private practice in Guilford, Connecticut. In keeping with behavioral optometry's tradition of bringing innovative vision care to other countries, Dr. Padula helped start a low vision clinic at the Zhongshan Eye Research Hospital in Guanhzhou, China, where he has been invited to direct services. (Chapter 9 has information on the pioneering work done in other countries).

Dr. Padula has authored publications and video tapes on low vision and in 1988, the OEP Foundation published his *A Behavioral Vision Approach for Persons with Physical Disabilities*. This is a valuable book, which discusses vision, how we use our vision system and the development of the visually impaired child. Subsequent chapters compare the perceptual development of the sighted and visually impaired child, the needs of the visually impaired, multihandicapped and brain injured, and the use of optical aids for those with low vision. Chapters on postural development and vision, and motor skills and vision have been contributed by specialists in fields such as occupational therapy and rehabilitation. The book is written primarily for the health practitioners involved in working with multihandicapped and visually impaired individuals, but it is definitely understandable to the general reader. It is a worthwhile addition to personal and public libraries for it opens new horizons in the field of treatment in cases of low vision, physical disability and traumatic injury.

A Three-year-old With Spastic Cerebral Palsy and Cortical Blindness

Somehow, parents with children diagnosed as multihandicapped must give the youngsters therapy and training for their physical and emotional needs. A three-year-old boy was brought to Dr. Padula for a low vision evaluation. He had spastic cerebral palsy, had been diagnosed as cortically blind and did not speak. The mother had been told by physicians that although the child could see a little, nothing could be done to help him improve his sight.

After a careful examination, Dr. Padula discovered that the boy did have some measure of visual function and the use of lenses to correct the child's farsightedness brought an increase in the vision system's functioning. Dr. Padula decided to prescribe the type of lenses used in the testing to be worn for one to two hours at a time. He also developed procedures for the parents to do with the boy. These included activities for tracking an object that the youngster held in his hand while a parent moved his hand until the boy began to initiate the movement himself and other procedures that encouraged the boy to reach and touch. Dr. Padula also developed a way for the parents to test the boy's clarity of sight daily.

Three months later, the mother returned with her son and reported substantial improvements in the child's behavior, awareness and posture. After the first week of wearing the glasses for the one to two hours daily, the boy stopped slumping in his chair while wearing the glasses. On this visit, Dr. Padula was able to measure significant improvements in the way the boy used his vision. The progress might have been slight in comparison with that of a sighted, nonhandicapped child but for this three-year-old, it represented major advancements in his use of vision.

A Lifelong Limp?

When Elizabeth came into Dr. Forkiotis' office, she dragged her left leg. Her parents told the receptionist that they had been referred to Dr. Forkiotis by the Gesell Institute. They explained that their ten-year-old daughter Elizabeth was diagnosed learning disabled and had repeated the first and third grades. Her teacher had commented that it was impossible to "get through to Elizabeth on any assignment." The parents had gone to Gesell because their daughter had been under the care of a neurologist and a rehabilitation center for the past four years, yet there had been little improvement. The neurological diagnosis was "contraction of the left leg." Elizabeth also had problems with her left ear and the quality of her hearing was poor. Gesell had recommended a complete visual analysis and had suggested also that vision therapy might be of value.

The family was originally from Puerto Rico and Spanish was their first language. Both parents, however, spoke fluent English, yet Elizabeth found it difficult to speak in English without doublechecking everything. She almost always confirmed her comments by speaking in Spanish to her parents. When Dr. Forkiotis asked the parents about this habit, they explained that they'd been told this was part of their daughter's learning problem. Elizabeth was not comfortable in school. She said she often had stomachaches, particularly at recess. Sometimes the chalkboard was not clear. She had to hold the books and papers close to her eyes but then her neck would ache. At home, she would feel hungry before meals, but not be able to eat when at the table. Her father told Dr. Forkiotis that he had checked to see if Elizabeth could follow a moving target and he found that the right eye followed the target, but the left eye didn't seem to move. At this stage, the family was considering placing Elizabeth in a private school, one where the classes were small.

When Dr. Forkiotis gave Elizabeth a visual analysis, he found that her color perception was completely accurate but very slow and the youngster had difficulty explaining what she saw. Further tests showed a tendency for her left eye to turn out. The most significant result of these tests was the differences in each eye's visual acuity. The left eye measured 20/80, while the right eye had a visual acuity of 20/120. This factor was a valuable clue which had not been evaluated until now.

Elizabeth found it impossible to complete all of the twenty-four tests in the analysis because her focusing and convergence-divergence abilities were so unstable. Each time she tried to complete any of the points in the testing, she would either have blurred vision or see double. Dr. Forkiotis asked the parents about Elizabeth's physical activities. He was told that because of the child's contracted leg, she never left the house. At school, she was always excused from sports or physical exercise. At this point, Dr. Forkiotis recommended weekly office visits and suggested that daily procedures done at home would be valuable. This led to the father working faithfully each night with Elizabeth for twenty minutes. Stress-reducing lenses for close work at school were prescribed.

Heartwarming Results

Three months later, Elizabeth had made great strides, literally, for her left leg was no longer contracted. The neurological stimulation from the therapy program had caused physiological changes. She was bike riding and roller skating--without lessons. She had gained two years in her classroom level.

When Dr. Forkiotis gave Elizabeth a second visual analysis, her reactions were totally different. She performed the visual tasks with ease and her visual function was of a high quality. Each eye had a visual acuity of 20/20 at both distance and close work--without any lens use. The next step was the recommendation that Elizabeth use her stress-relieving lenses for all close work, as a precaution.

The parents were overjoyed at the changes brought about by the therapy. They were incensed by the inadequate but costly care they had received before they found Dr. Forkiotis, because it had robbed their daughter of so much in her childhood. They moved back to Puerto Rico. They took with them a happy child who had been able to outstrip a crippling physical infirmity and learning disability with the help of a drug-free, surgery-free program of optometric vision therapy.

Chapter 7

The Team Approach: Repairing the Damage

When youngsters or adults with learning or behavior difficulties are helped by optometric vision therapy to develop efficient vision systems, that's often only the first step along the way to helping them develop fully productive lives. Frequently, these individuals have not developed efficient skills in reading and writing. Children may be behind their grade levels in most studies. Proper study habits are foreign to them. They lack organizational skills. Often, they have mild to severe emotional problems which may range from feelings of unworthiness to rebellious rage.

It is one situation to fix the cause of these problems. It is another to repair the damage. Often, the repairs call for a team approach. In addition to the optometrist who provides vision therapy, a team can include experts in the fields of education, psychology, nutrition, occupational therapy and child development. You can find addresses and information in Chapter 9.

Many private practitioners will also suggest other therapies when appropriate.

Let's Help Jane and John Read

Literacy is a basic indication of how well we function as individuals and as a nation. In the book, *Megatrends*, John Naisbitt says that the Carnegie Council of Policy Studies in Higher Education estimated that in the 1980s, the number of functional illiterates in the United States ranged from 18-64 million. Even more discouraging is the growing number of high school dropouts.

Naisbitt points out that "in the bellwether state of California, the dropout rate increased 83 percent during the 1970s and now is three times the national average." Other states, including Ohio, New York and Wisconsin have reported both increased dropouts and chronic absenteeism, which usually leads to higher dropout rates.

Studies by optometrists around the country, in particular Dr. Kaseno in California and Dr. Zaba in Virginia, prove the connection between vision imbalances and learning difficulties.

Optometric vision therapy can help change literacy levels by changing the underlying vision imbalances that trigger difficulties in learning.

Networking by Practitioners

The linking of health practitioners in a referral and support network is valuable. Practitioners who network view such referral as a means of providing their patients with the most comprehensive health care possible, as the following case histories show.

Tutoring--What Sort Is Needed?

Anne Bowden is a youngster whose experience illustrates how vital tutoring may be once optometric vision therapy has helped remedy vision imbalances. Which tutoring to select is not always obvious. In Anne's case, it took careful evaluation of where she needed help with her schoolwork.

Anne was treated by Dr. David Friedel of Tucson, Arizona, whose practice is devoted to optometric vision therapy. In 1983, when Anne was in fourth grade, her parents were desperate to find help for their daughter, who was reading way below grade level. Their two other children had no problems and all three youngsters had similar IQs. Anne's mother, Emily, specializes in teaching the learning disabled, yet she had spent many frustrating months trying to tutor her own daughter. All her efforts were unsuccessful.

"She flip-flopped words and was not making any progress. We'd been told she was all sorts of things, from dyslexic to learning disabled. Her sight had been tested and we'd been assured it was fine," Anne's mother says. "Each year, I'd tried a different ophthalmologist, starting in first grade. By fourth grade, we were on the fourth, who repeated what all the others had said. Anne had better than 20/20 sight. He assured me her eyes were not the cause of her learning difficulties but that emotional problems were. He recommended Anne be given Ritalin, an amphetamine which stimulates the central nervous system. I was shocked. I'd worked with youngsters on Ritalin and I know its results. It's a pretty serious drug.

"Just after that visit, which was pretty devastating, a neighbor was at the house. She sat at the table with Anne, helping her read a simple primer. Anne, who is very bright, was desperate to read and she'd memorized the simple text. The neighbor noticed Anne's eyes were making jerky movements as they moved across the page. Turning to me she said, 'Have you seen Doctor Friedel? My son had the same jerky eye movements and he was helped by this doctor.'

"My first reaction was one of hysterical rejection. No! Not another doctor. Her eyes were fine, better than 20/20. Then, the next morning, I woke up and thought about it and realized I was hearing something new. Eye movements. I thought, what do I have to lose? It might help. I called Dr. Friedel and I have to admit, I burst into tears. The nervous strain was so great, it had built up over so long. He took time out to talk to me on the phone. A few days later, when I took Anne in, she and I both broke down and cried. We were that desperate for help.

"Once vision therapy started, Anne did the home procedures Dr. Friedel gave her religiously but her school progress was slow. After a few months of the therapy, we started tutoring. The tutor discovered the NIM program [see Appendix 5 for a brief explanation of NIM, neurological impress remedial reading technique]. Anne's schoolwork began to improve. I realized two things were happening: her vision system was responding to the special training with Dr. Friedel and the correct type of tutoring was making the difference in helping Anne close the gap on her academic loss. Then we found she didn't know her phonics, so the tutor started with them. That coupled with the NIM program and the ongoing vision therapy at home made a dramatic difference.

"Anne jumped her reading level about six months' worth. The school did not think she could graduate from fifth grade but she did. They'd never seen a child turn around like this. Anne wanted so much to be like everyone else, and once Dr. Friedel had taught her how to bring some balance to her vision system, she could also handle the tutoring. Remember, I've worked with dozens of youngsters in need of tutoring, and I realized something very important when I looked back at the past years."

Tutoring Hopeless If Vision Inadequate

"My daughter needed tutoring desperately by the time she had reached the fourth grade but until she had optometric vision therapy, she could never benefit from tutoring. For instance, she was a math whiz under the right circumstances. When someone read complicated math word problems to her, she could do them in her head. Otherwise, she couldn't handle math. So her frustration with math was high. Once she could tackle reading, a result of combining the vision therapy and the right tutoring, she could settle down and at least approach her schoolwork on a reasonable level."

Anne's mother also points out that it is important that the school know the child has a vision imbalance. "That's another aspect of the situation. You have to help educate the teachers. Certain things are better handled certain ways with a youngster like Anne. Even something that seems as simple as not having the other children call her dummy and call out words when she's trying to read." A year after Anne had completed her vision therapy, her mother still has vivid memories of the sharpness of the family's despair before meeting Dr. Friedel-- and the incredible change the therapy and correct tutoring made to Anne and the family.

Schools Are On The Team

An optometrist whose work with schools spans decades, Dr. John Streff, co-founder and former director of the S. A. NOEL Center in Lancaster, Ohio, has been involved with creating vision programs for school systems since the 1960s, when he was head of the Department of Visual Research at Connecticut's Gesell Institute. Widely regarded as one of behavioral optometry's august deans, Dr. Streff organized programs for schools in Vermont and Connecticut backed by a Federal Title I grant. By placing children according to their developmental rather than chronological age, his programs helped reduce the schools' needs and costs for special services and remedial reading.

The center was named to honor the memories and work of Drs. A. M. Skeffington and E. B. Alexander, founders of the Optometric Extension Program Foundation. Ohio was deliberately chosen because Dr. Streff felt that Lancaster, which is centrally located in the country, was a good test market. It has a reasonably sized population of some 45,000, is near a large metropolitan center and has a private school (parochial) which had expressed a commitment to the center's program of education and research to establish a clinical and educational facility. The center, which opened in 1980, ran until 1989. It began with a staff of three individuals whose backgrounds were different but complementary: Sr. Barbara Jinks, an educator, Bruce Wolff, an optometrist known for his innovative clinical work and Dr. Streff.

The center ran a community service program which was available to each child who entered kindergarten. Some 90 percent of the enrollment were in the program and were followed through third grade. The center documented the changes after lenses were put on the youngsters. Overactive children calmed down, passive youngsters became more involved. The lenses changed the children's abilities to sit and learn. The center also had a clinic which handled over one hundred vision therapy patients each week; some were children in the school study, others were patients referred from outside sources. Dr. Streff explains that lenses are a tool for the type of environment we have today.

"Youngsters playing baseball wear gloves to protect their hands, not because there's something wrong with their hands. It's the same with the type of lenses we use, they are protective or developmental--and very necessary in a society that requires so much close work. I wonder if people had as much trouble accepting shoes when they started wearing them?"

Collaboration With Physical Therapists and Psychologists

An article in the April 1966 issue of *Woman's Day*, "Your Child's Vision Can Be Improved," by Charles Cerami, discussed the history of Virginia, a retarded four-year-old. She was considered a hopeless mental cripple. Virginia spent all her day standing over a toy ironing board, endlessly pressing the same piece of cloth. Her vision had deteriorated until she could hardly see a foot in front of her face. Concerned that the child was going blind, her parents took her to Dr. Morton Davis, a practitioner of optometric vision therapy in Bethesda, Maryland.

Virginia's parents agreed to let psychologists and physical therapists take part in planning a treatment program with Dr. Davis. The Physical Education Department at the University of Maryland gave the child exercises to develop coordination. Work on a trampoline was especially stressed, for this forces many systems of the body to work at the same time. The psychologists instructed Virginia's parents to make the child look and reach just beyond her normal range for anything she wanted. It was necessary to handle this aspect of the therapy carefully so as not to frustrate the youngster. Eventually, Virginia had made enough progress so that she could work with some of the simpler vision therapy procedures. As a result, Dr. Davis was able to reverse Virginia's nearsightedness. In fact, he reduced it by some 60 percent. The upshot of the teamwork was that Virginia can no longer be diagnosed retarded. Her IQ score had climbed to the low normal range.

"It's hard for me to read and write--why?"

Matthew, a thirty-one-year-old man, was referred to the Learning Disabilities Unit at the State University of New York, State College of Optometry. Dr. Rochelle Mozlin, an assistant clinical professor at the College of Optometry, wrote about Matthew in the January 1985 *Optometry Times* column "My Most Interesting Case." Matthew "had always had difficulty with reading, writing and spelling and wanted to know the reason for his difficulties and what could be done to help him improve his skills. Matthew had many of the signs and symptoms that suggest a visual problem, including difficulty in concentrating, poor comprehension, the use of a finger to keep his place and giving up after fifteen minutes.

"A psychoeducational evaluation showed Matthew to be a bright man with a severe learning disability. Since his academic skills were barely adequate for survival in the business world, it was recommended that Matthew begin to work with a learning disabilities specialist to develop reading and writing skills," wrote Dr. Mozlin.

Dr. Mozlin gave Matthew a visual analysis as part of his evaluation to determine if his learning problems included a visual component. Matthew did indeed have significant visual imbalances, the most serious were that his eyes did not team well and his accommodative skill, or ability to change focus, was extremely poor.

The next step was a conference between Matthew, the psychologist who had made the psychoeducational evaluation, and optometrist Dr. Mozlin. Priorities were listed. Dr. Mozlin says, "We developed a plan and a timetable for an effective remediation of his learning disability. The first phase was a program of vision therapy. Goals of the therapeutic program, which were established at the outset, were to improve the quality of Matthew's vision imbalances. I explained to Matthew that the vision therapy per se would not solve his reading problems. Rather, it would eliminate his symptoms and permit him to perform nearpoint activities with greater comfort for longer periods of time, facilitating an improved response to reading and other instruction that was to follow.

"The first month of therapy brought rapid progress. Matthew improved his visual abilities considerably and changed the quality of his vision functioning from low to close to average. He had glasses for reading, to help his system function adequately while doing close work. After four months of weekly visits to the clinic, Matthew stopped that phase of the program and moved to the next: working with a learning disabilities specialist. He was now able to read for longer periods with greater comfort and understanding."

A test made after four months of vision therapy showed that Matthew's reading performance had improved considerably. Although another course of vision therapy would help Matthew improve even more, at this stage in the program it was necessary that Matthew work with the learning disabilities specialist to develop reading and writing skills. Dr. Mozlin felt that further vision therapy would be of value at a later date, perhaps in a year.

Dr. Mozlin wrote that this case was of particular interest to her because it demonstrated that the treatment of learning disabilities is multidisciplinary. The role of optometry in Matthew's case was significant but it was strengthened by the cooperation with psychology and special education.

"By establishing priorities and developing a multifaceted program for the treatment of Matthew's complex problem, a team of professionals, working together, was able to change this man's life."

Optometry and Ophthalmology Interact

The case history of Peter River is an outstanding example of teamwork between optometry and ophthalmology. It is also the heartwrenching story of someone who was told he was going blind and nothing could be done to reverse the situation. Peter was forty-nine when he first was examined by Dr. Tirsa Quinones of New Haven, Connecticut, in March of 1982. In the previous six to eight months, he had suffered a rapid loss of central visual acuity first in the right eye and then in the left eye. Apart from his visual problem, the patient was in perfect health. By the time he reached Dr. Quinones, he had undergone extensive medical analyses, including a series of ophthalmological and neurological studies in Puerto Rico, Florida and Maryland.

The conclusion of the various teams was that the loss of visual acuity was due to an optic nerve atrophy identified as Leber's Disease. This condition affects young people (eighteen to twenty-three years of age) and usually there is a family history. This individual did not match these characteristics. Nor did his clinical symptoms match the disease's syndromes completely. Yet the diagnosis was that soon Peter would be left with little or no sight, virtually blind, as the condition deteriorated. A traveling salesman, Peter was severely hindered by the sudden visual loss. He was not able to drive or perform the bulk of his work without assistance. Quite naturally, he was feeling extremely tense and frustrated, additional pressure on a vision system clearly imbalanced and dysfunctioning.

At this stage, a mutual acquaintance recommended Dr. Quinones to Peter. Before she started optometric care, Dr. Quinones suggested that Peter have a complete workup with a local practitioner, Dr. Rocko Fasanella, a prominent ophthalmologist with whom she works very closely. After extensive tests, Dr. Fasanella concluded that the case did not present a picture of Leber's Optic Atrophy. In his opinion, the condition may have been related to vascular problems in the carotid system. Vascular studies were then performed by a team of physicians at the Yale-New Haven Hospital. The results did not show any evidence of major vascular obstructions and the diagnosis was "optic nerve atrophy of unknown etiology."

When Dr. Quinones started her evaluations of the way Peter's vision system functioned, she also consulted with Dr. William Padula, because he specializes in low vision. His evaluation showed a definite loss of visual acuity, but at the same time, the visual fields showed significant intact peripheral areas. This was important, since Dr. Quinones hoped to stimulate as much peripheral visual use as possible so that Peter could continue to get around. At this stage, he had little trouble walking around, although he did have some balance problems, something which does occur when there is loss of central or peripheral vision. His main difficulty was perception of visual detail.

Telescopic lenses and magnifiers were tried for activities such as watching television and looking at small details close up. Peter found these devices frustrating, since it was hard for him to accept his vision difficulties. This is not uncommon in such cases. Dr. Padula also suggested a nutritional analysis and an elimination of fats and cholesterol, including the reduction and ultimately the complete elimination of red meat intake. At this stage, Dr. Quinones began optometric vision therapy designed both to maintain peripheral visual activity and also to relieve as much visual stress as possible. The therapy included balance activities and a great deal of work with yoke prisms. Lenses which include prisms are used to stimulate all areas of the peripheral retina while the individual is engaged in visual activities such as peripheral awareness activities. Dr. Quinones emphasized therapy that built easy eye movement control; she deemphasized activities that included small detail. By the second week of optometric vision therapy, which Peter did virtually each day at home, a minor miracle occurred. He called Dr. Quinones to tell her that while shaving, he was able to see his beard in the mirror. Immediately, Dr. Quinones knew that some of the central visual acuity was being activated.

For the next three weeks, Peter visited Dr. Quinones at her New Haven office while continuing his home procedures. Then he returned to Puerto Rico. Dr. Quinones had designed a full program of daily home procedures for Peter since he would be living so far away. His wife was very supportive and helpful, and they followed the recommendations faithfully. About two months after Peter and his wife had returned to Puerto Rico, Dr. Quinones received a call from his wife. The news was excellent. Peter was able to drive again. His central visual acuity had improved significantly. He was able to read signs and see traffic lights, and he was slowly increasing his work schedule. The home program was continued for several more months and Dr. Quinones incorporated a prismatic component into the patient's regular lens prescription that would continue to reduce visual stress and stimulate easy seeing.

Peter returned to New Haven for an evaluation in 1985. When he had first been examined by Dr. Quinones in 1982, his visual acuity was 20/200 in the right eye and 20/100 in the left eye. Now, although he had low acuity in the right eye, his left eye acuity was 20/40 and he had an acuity of 20/40 with both eyes, a phenomenal improvement. Equally significant was the fact that Peter was able to carry a full work schedule. Naturally, he had lost the tenseness and frustration which had developed at the prospect of going blind. In her report, Dr. Quinones wrote:

"This is an example of a case which had been misdiagnosed as optic nerve atrophy of the sort that would cause irreversible visual acuity loss. A team of an ophthalmologist, a low vision specialist and a behavioral optometrist worked together and ultimately, after all ophthalmological roots were explored, the case was dealt with by behavioral optometry. The patient came to my office for 5 weeks then worked at home, in Puerto Rico, for some 18 months.

"Lenses and special prisms were used to stimulate and maintain peripheral awareness, which will cause the relaxation of visual perception. Work in the area of eye movement control, multisensory integration and accommodative facility was extremely important in relieving the intense visual stress pattern the patient showed. He was able to improve his vision significantly enough to resume normal functioning and to do what was important to him.

"This case shows the value of a functional approach in cases of low vision, although results may not be as dramatic in all cases as in this case. We have seen many low vision cases where optometric vision therapy is extremely helpful in that it allows the individuals to use the vision available to them in an easier, more productive and less stressful way."

Fine-tuning the Stars

Professional athletes whose achievement levels are high and who often have excellent vision skills, are nonetheless enthusiastic users of sports vision therapy. Among them, super-achievers such as tennis champion Virginia Wade; 20-game winner Bucky Dent; teams that have dominated their sports like the Dallas Cowboys and the New York Yankees and, not least, the US Olympic Gold volleyball and Bronze field hockey teams. All have described significant improvements in their play and in their lives.

When the US men's volleyball team zapped the team from Brazil three games to none to win its first-ever Olympic gold medal in 1984, Bob Sanet, O.D., of San Diego was in the audience cheering hard. Dr. Sanet said, "I can't claim I was responsible for the team's success. They played phenomenally well. But I do feel that I had a part in the victory."

It all began in March 1983, when three members of the Sports Vision Section of the American Optometric Association, Drs. Don Getz, Garry Etting and Bob Sanet, were sent by officials at the Olympic Training Center in Colorado Springs to screen members of the men's volleyball team. Tests showed that four of the athletes were performing well below the level of their team mates, despite 20/20 sight. The four had trouble moving their eyes smoothly when their bodies were off balance. One actually took his eyes off the ball at those times.

Dr. Sanet explains that athletes will often compensate for a visual deficiency by relying on another sense. Experienced volleyball players can tell by the sound of the ball how fast it is traveling. This may be compensating for an inability to track or follow the ball visually. The compensating takes its toll as the competition becomes tougher. By the time an athlete reaches the Olympics, the split second it takes to compensate for a visual deficiency may mean the difference between a gold medal and sixth place. Over the next year, whenever the team was in town. Dr. Sanet worked with Chris Marlowe, Craig Buck, Steve Salmons and Rich Duwelius, giving them vision therapy activities to improve their game. At first, the players were reluctant to try the activities. Assistant Coach Tony Crabb explained that topnotch athletes are often wary of trying something new for fear it will ruin a winning formula.

The first who did try, Salmons, made slow progress at the beginning but kept to it. His hitting percentage showed a steady increase, growing from 26 per cent on an April tour to Cuba to 55 per cent on a September tour to Japan. On the Japan tour, he was named the most valuable player. The impressive statistics convinced the three others to concentrate on the training. Buck, who at first was the least enthusiastic, improved the most, Dr. Sanet reported. "He played beautifully in the finals," the optometrist added. Buck summed up the athletes' feelings about vision therapy. "The world looks different to me now. I never realized there was so much depth."

The four volleyball players who received the extensive vision care had hitting percentages in the 20 percent range when vision sessions began. After the therapy, their hitting percentages moved to 40-50 percent.

Their vision analyses showed at the start that all four players, despite 20/20 sight, had problems with depth perception, tracking moving objects and keeping both eyes "turned in" at all times. Coach Crabb said their charts looked like seismographs. "I wish they'd all go to vision therapy. I think it can only help. And I think they need it."

Dr. Etting and Dr. Getz, who created the program for our Olympic volleyballers, had both worked with top athletes. They helped develop vision therapy programs for the 1980 and 1984 US Olympic teams and participated in screening programs at the National Sports Festival in 1979, 1981 and 1982.

Nothing Succeeds Like Success

The Yankee baseball organization demonstrated their support of and belief in optometric vision therapy by helping Dr. Donald Teig of Connecticut produce a thirty-second television public service message in the late 1970s. Dr. Teig had worked with several of the Yankees on a variety of vision programs, including one for batters. He had proved the value of vision training in terms of batting averages and throwing strikes. As a result, Yankee catcher Fran Healy, first baseman Chris Chambliss and ace relief pitcher Sparky Lyle all appeared in the TV message.

Racing champions like motorcyclist Kenny Roberts who are looking at million-dollar incomes have discovered that optometric vision therapy is one way to gain a real competitive edge. Dr. Etting has designed a two-hour series of more than sixty tests to measure sports vision skills and to determine how well a person like Roberts uses visual information. In 1983, at the instigation of *Cycle* magazine, five of the world's top motorcycle champions underwent Etting's daunting battery of vision analysis tests. They included Mike Bell, Bruce Penhall, Eddie Lawson, Chriss Heisser and Mike Haller. The results, as you might expect from their previous records of superior performances, showed superior vision systems. Few vision imbalances were detected. In fact, Mike Bell, a Supercross champion recognized as one of the best motorcross riders in the world, has such a superior system he actually beat the machine that tested for peripheral vision.

Hole in One

Val Skinner, professional woman golfer is very articulate about the way optometric vision therapy helped her improve her game. When she was twenty, the golfer went to see Dr. Sue Lowe, a behavioral optometrist in Laramie, Wyoming, at the suggestion of a friend. After two years of watching her golf game deteriorate, Val Skinner's reaction to the suggestion was, "Why not give optometric vision therapy a shot? I was waking up every morning with headaches and grinding my teeth. My father is my coach, and he was very supportive about trying the therapy. At first, it was really hard to convince me that anything was wrong with my eyes. I couldn't understand how, if my eyes were so bad, I could ever have become a professional athlete."

After an initial visual exam, Dr. Lowe told Ms. Skinner that on a scale of one to ten, Val's visual skills rated a two. This, with the explanation from Dr. Lowe of why Val's vision system was so out of whack, was enough motivation for the young golfer to commit herself to two months of intensive, daily therapy with Dr. Lowe. Most of us are not able (or willing) to plunge so extensively into therapy, but from the viewpoint of a professional athlete it's plain common sense. The sooner you can regain the performance needed in your sport, the sooner you are back in competition.

"As an athlete, vision therapy helped me," says Val Skinner. "I can't put a percentage on the exact amount, but my game is far superior now than it had been before I took the therapy with Dr. Lowe. Tangible proof came early on, when my headaches disappeared and I stopped grinding my teeth. Just as importantly, vision therapy helped me as an individual."

Ms. Skinner practices visualization skills quite often and has learned to allow her eyes to lead her body.

"The therapy taught me to look at the target and let my body go with my eyes. My work with Dr. Lowe was nonstop for several months. I had the experience of making my own visual progress and also seeing others go through the training and make phenomenal changes. That had a tremendous impact on me. I hope that someday this type of optometric care will be available and used by everyone."

Shocking Surprise

You can be a fine performer at sports, confident in your abilities. You can consider yourself quite normal, with no vision problems. You may not wear glasses or contact lenses or, if you do, you have the idea they're taking care of all your vision needs. Then you can undergo a vision analysis and face a shocking surprise. Writer Jeffrey Hansen describes how he felt when interviewing Dr. Etting.

"He left me wondering whether to laugh, cry or punch his lights out."

Hansen had visited Dr. Etting after hearing the tale of a former patient of the optometrist's, a baseball player who, after nearly slipping into oblivion, took vision therapy and then was drafted by the majors. As a writer in search of a story, Hansen readily accepted Dr. Etting's offer to put him through a series of a half dozen tests to illustrate the various facets of vision analysis and care. Hansen was skeptical.

"After all," he reasoned. "I have 20/20 sight." What could the optometrist tell him that he could make into a story. To his chagrin, Hansen discovered that he "had not the barest minimum of depth perception.

"My eyes didn't work together as a team. Under stress, my eyes constricted into tunnel vision. Suddenly, I remembered and began to understand puzzling childhood problems."

Reading had literally given him headaches as a teenager. Sports were also difficult. As an adult, he had become an enthusiastic amateur motorcycle racer but he crashed a lot in desert races. On a closed motorcycle track, although never winning races, Hansen was more successful and rarely crashed. Why? Dr. Etting explained that Hansen's vision system could pick up and react to vision clues that didn't change on the closed motorcycle track. On the wide open and varied desert terrain, there were few clues for his vision system to pick up and react to quickly enough for him to handle changes. So he would sometimes crash.

"The sudden understanding of my limitations didn't make them any easier to face," writes Hansen. After undertaking a specially designed program that gave him sixteen different vision therapy procedures to do at home and similar activities in Dr. Etting's office, Hansen found his life changing. "One day," he writes, "I had the pure and sudden joy of walking out of the office door and seeing the world for the very first time in 3-D." The way most people see the world!

The Moment of Truth

John Fulton is one of only a few Americans who have become full-fledged matadors and have practiced the art of bullfighting in the arenas of Spain and Mexico. Fulton is also an artist who deals mainly in subjects related to the bullring. You can see his work in a gallery he runs in Majorca. He also collaborated with James Michener on the book *Iberia*.

Fulton was in his forties when chance put him together with Dr. Carl W. Childress, an optometrist from Texas who was in Spain fulfilling his US Naval Reserve obligations. When

Dr. Childress gave Fulton a vision analysis, he discovered the Yanqui matador had a surprising array of vision imbalances. Fulton had mentioned to Dr. Childress that his bullfighting colleagues had often commented on the greater than normal distance Fulton kept between himself and the bull during his capework in preparation for the kill. Far from this being a lack of courage, Dr. Childress found that Fulton's vision imbalances made it impossible for him to judge with any accuracy where the rampaging bull was positioned at many critical moments in his encounters.

"Like most people," Dr. Childress recalls, "John didn't recognize that he had vision problems."

The vision analysis revealed that Fulton's eyes were not teaming. This led to occasional double vision and alternating suppression. In other words, first one eye, then the other would shut down. This caused inaccurate depth perception. Not the situation of choice when confronting a bull. Fulton was so impressed by the optometrist's analysis that eventually he traveled to the doctor's Texas office for further testing and a course of optometric vision therapy.

A series of procedures was designed for Fulton, and after his return to Spain and a period of devoting himself to this practice, Fulton was able to write to Dr. Childress with a good report. "I no longer have any headaches and I'm not aware of blurred or double vision." He also commented, "I still think that what you did for me is some kind of miracle and have been talking to everyone about it and given your address to some."

Attitudes and Perception

A youngster who has little problem rattling off the letters on an optometrist's eye chart but who has a visual disorder may misread her family to the point of seeing instability where it doesn't exist.

This is the conclusion of a study by Dr. Joel Zaba, an optometrist in Norfolk, Virginia, and his associate, psychologist

Gary Bachara, Ph.D., of Wilson, North Carolina. The study is one in a series in which the two researchers have linked visual perception problems to learning disabilities, behavioral problems and juvenile delinquency.

"Twenty-twenty eyesight does not guarantee perfect perception," says Dr. Zaba. "Even if a child is not nearsighted or farsighted, we cannot conclude that his vision is good. Our study shows that children with visual problems tend to see instability in their families, whether or not the families are unstable."

The study, funded by the American Optometric Foundation, looked at 270 children divided into three equal groups of ninety. One group included children with visual perception problems. Another group was receiving professional help for psychological or behavioral problems. The remaining subjects made up the control group. A story in the *Virginian-Pilot* of July 6, 1987, "Eye disorders affect perception of family," by Joseph Cosco, reported that "Each child was asked to create a 'family kinetic drawing,' a portrait of himself and his family performing some activity. Psychologist Bachara then interpreted the drawings by using a standardized scoring system."

Dr. Bachara found that thirty-one of the children in the group with visual perception problems saw instability in their families, compared with fifty-seven in the group that was receiving professional psychological help and nineteen in the control group. He theorized that the visually-impaired children were seeing instability because of feelings that their learning problems were creating upheaval in the family.

The psychologist commented that "usually, the mother and father argue about how strict they should be with these youngsters, who are generally bright but not performing up to expectations." Naturally, the situation leads to a vicious cycle. When a youngster believes the family is unstable, this probably adds to the child's feeling of insecurity. This in turn will create additional stress which will make it hard to cope with learning or behavior problems.

Fortunately, although many of the children with perception problems were misreading their home lives and believing there was instability, they did not feel rejected by their families, according to Dr. Bachara's interpretation of the drawings. Only nine of the children expressed feelings of rejection, compared with twenty-seven in the group receiving professional help and eight in the control group. This was the only surprise to the psychologist, who had theorized at first that the group with visual perception problems might feel rejected. He suggested that perhaps they weren't feeling rejected because their parents obviously were concerned enough about the children's problems to begin seeking outside help.

Are There Answers?

A previous study by Dr. Zaba, also funded by a research grant from the American Optometric Foundation, investigated the emotional considerations of children with learning-related visual problems. 400 youngsters, 200 with learning-related vision imbalances and 200 without, were studied.

The results showed that when vision therapy helped overcome vision problems, the emotional problems decreased almost by half.

In the paper, "Visual and Perceptual Motor Training: A Psychologist's Viewpoint," part of a presentation read before the 1975 Annual Virginia Association for Children with Learning Disabilities, Dr. Bachara said that the question plaguing psychologists, educators, psychiatrists, or anyone who deals with children who have learning problems which are visual or visual-perceptual in nature is: To refer or not to refer.

"Anyone dealing with children in the mental health field is therefore confronted with the dilemma of appropriate diagnosis and remediation of the children's learning problem," Dr.

Bachara commented. He went on to explain that he became aware of controversy surrounding the use of optometric visual therapy only after he had adopted it as part of a multidisciplinary team approach at his counseling facility. They made extensive referrals for visual training whenever desirable, in conjunction with other modes of psychiatric care, educational remediation, hospitalization, and neurological evaluation. Intrigued by the inconsistency of the many studies critical of optometric vision therapy, the psychologist joined forces with Dr. Zaba for the specific purpose of studying, researching and publishing reliable material.

Dr. Bachara wrote that in his research, "one cannot help but find various attacks, opinionated rebuttals and verbal accusations. Many of these articles are heavily loaded with opinion and emotionally laden accusations. Many of the studies on learning-disabled children, who were not operationally defined, submitted them to perceptual-motor training for a short period of time and measured their reading ability afterward. Upon finding no increase in the reading level, they concluded that perceptual-motor training was of no use.

"Many times a misconstrued idea of the purpose of perceptual-motor and visual-motor training is that this training improves reading, which is erroneous. The training programs are geared to improve readiness to learn and readiness to read.

"As Zaba stated, vision therapy is similar to insulin. He drew this corollary. 'We would not give insulin to all children and expect them to be functioning better. It would only help the children who are diabetic and require it.' Similarly, he says, vision therapy will only help the child who needs it and not all children, and certainly not all learning-disabled children."

In "Psychological Effects of Visual Training," a joint paper by Drs. Bachara and Zaba, the authors once again stressed that a multidisciplinary approach toward learning problems is essential. This paper was on a study which examined the fact that there are more indicators of emotional involvement in the drawings of children who have learning and visual perceptual problems than there are in the drawings of those not experiencing these difficulties. Vision therapy twice weekly for four to six months brought significant changes in the drawings of the youngsters in the study.

"In the initial study comparing Groups A and B...the drawings pointed to the presence of feelings of inadequacy and a general sense of insecurity and helplessness. The results of this study indicate a decrease in emotional involvement after a visual training program. It appears that for children who are experiencing minor emotional difficulties associated with learning difficulties, forms of academic therapy and educational remediation, such as visual perceptual training, are very therapeutic in alleviating some of their minor stress. This is not to indicate that visual training or academic therapy be a substitute for psychotherapy or any other psychiatric intervention for those children requiring psychiatric care."

Papers by Drs. Bachara and Zaba have been published in *Academic Therapy,* the *Journal of Learning Disabilities* and optometric publications. Dr. Zaba, who is the visual consultant to the Norfolk Public School system, has lectured throughout the United States and has appeared on several television programs, including NBC's "Today" show and the USA cable network program, "Alive and Well." Dr. Bachara has served as a consultant for many health-related programs and associations dealing with children and learning disabilities.

Child Abuse and School Dropouts

The work of Charles Blaise and his ceaseless efforts to improve the quality of vision care in his home state of Louisiana eventually resulted in Act No. 156 being passed in that state. This act provides for a vision-hearing evaluation by a behavioral optometrist and an audiologist in addition to the usual medical examination of a juvenile, which may be ordered by the court. Mr. Blaise touches on another aspect of the effect of vision imbalances in a letter to the *Times Picayune.*

In "Eliminating Child Abuse," which was published on May 16, 1984, Mr. Blaise wrote that he and "a group of dedicated optometrists and legislators have done extensive research into the cause not only of child abuse but also of delinquency, school dropouts and learning disorders." Mr. Blaise writes that after it was determined that contributing factors are malfunctions in the sensory, visual and hearing systems of many of the abused and abusers, the landmark legislation gained its necessary support.

A Richness of Collaboration

The women and men who practice this therapy are noted for developing astonishingly diverse collaborations. Education, psychiatry, psychology, sports, pediatrics, geriatrics, nutrition, practitioners of optometric vision therapy interact with a wide variety of disciplines. It's only natural that their work reflects the interests of the practitioners. The following is a scant sampling of the diversity.

Dr. Ben Lane of Lake Hiawatha, New Jersey, is known internationally for his groundbreaking work with nutrition, health and vision; Dr. Martin Kane of Philadelphia, Pennsylvania, in addition to a private practice has held faculty appointments at Drexel, Antioch and Pennsylvania State universities, regularly teaching graduate and undergraduate courses in early childhood education and human learning and development. Dr. Kane was editor of the *Journal of Optometric Vision Development* for several decades, for which he was awarded national prizes; Dr. Walter Kaplan of Gaithersburg, Maryland, has been involved with multidisciplinary health care delivery (HMO) in addition to his private practice and has also been a prolific contributor to optometric journals for many years.

Dr. Robert Pepper of Oregon spent twenty years developing a program to encourage vision, movement, speech, hearing and learning specialists to coordinate team efforts to develop human potential. The main focus of his work is the enhancement of kinesthetic processing. Dr. Pepper eventually broadened the use of this program from his professional optometric practice to include the high achiever, particularly the skilled athlete. In partnership with Dr. Winnefred L. Wyckoff, Associate Professor of Physical Education at Oregon State University, Dr. Pepper worked with coaches and athletes of the NBA Portland Trailblazers and conducted workshops and clinics for high school coaches and players. The program is also available for college and university coaches.

The Cheshire Study and the Coronado Project

These are two of the studies that show the value of using optometric vision therapy in the school setting. The study of 822 children (sixth graders) in Cheshire, Connecticut, started in the 1960s under the guidance of Dr. John Streff. Students from the School of Architecture and Design at Yale University, under the direction of Professor Felix Drewry, recommended and constructed physical environmental changes. These varied from changing room lighting and designing classroom equipment to physical changes.

The youngsters in the test were all from Cheshire, while the control groups were from a neighboring school system. A motor-sensory development and problem-solving activities program started in February 1966, with a pilot program in the second grade. Studies continued through the mid-1970s. The benefits of the Cheshire studies were varied. It yielded valuable information on the development of nearsightedness. Score levels in the Cheshire schools changed as a result of the program, while those of the control groups remained the same. The program also proved helpful to those teachers who were supportive of the program and who incorporated suggestions on work habits into their daily routine. The school systems saved on the costs of remedial programs, also.

In *Stop School Failure,* which Harper & Row published in 1972, Dr. Streff devoted Chapter 12 to a careful evaluation of the Cheshire study. "It was never our intent merely to carry out optometric vision therapy in the school." He explains that one half hour a day was set aside to involve children in activities that encouraged movement, communication among themselves, group interaction and figuring things out. "Yes, a program like this can change things in the classroom, but it depends on the teacher," he concluded. He wrote that about a third of the teachers changed their teaching style dramatically; another third made significant changes in style and approach, while the remaining third made from "some" to "slight" change.

The Cheshire program was begun at the initiative of Mrs. Gwynette Caruthers, the school psychologist for the Cheshire Public Schools, who visited the Gesell Institute to broach plans for the study. Mrs. Caruthers, who had had extensive classroom experience before becoming a psychologist, was disturbed about what was happening to children in the schools. She noted that many behavior problems first appeared, or were intensified, after children enter school. She was also concerned that the quality of classroom activity or special education programs often failed to meet the needs of the children. She went to Gesell for she was aware of their success in solving some of the kinds of problems about which she was concerned.

It makes sense now, decades later, to offer the programs based on the concepts of optometric vision therapy to school youngsters as early as possible. Why wait for them to have problems with their work that force them into remedial education, or cause them to drop out of school or become delinquents? Isn't it also equally appropriate to inform teachers of these programs in college?

The Coronado Project began in the Coronado Unified School District, California, in 1970 under the direction of Dr. W. Keith Wilson, Jay D. Mack, Ed.D., and Ann H. Breslauer, B.A. Its aim was both to work with a carefully selected group of twenty-seven youngsters (kindergarten through sixth grade); children already in optometric vision therapy or with strabismus or amblyopia were excluded. The project also offered teacher training and parent education. Staff included a director, a teacher, teacher's aide, educational consultant, optometric consultant, school nurse, psychologist, speech teacher and project evaluator. An advisory council of a classroom teacher, parents of two project pupils, a pediatrician, an optometrist, and a representative from the San Diego County Department of Education Special Education Services, and a project teacher and project director was established for advisory and community liaison.

In a report published in 1975 by the Optometric Extension Program Foundation, the conclusions were listed as good. "The project group showed marked improvement on each of the five areas of training aimed at improving visual efficiency. Academic gains were evidenced by improved test performance in all three academic areas measured. Spelling and arithmetic gains were actually better than those of reading when the number of pupils making a gain of one year is considered. Over two third of the project group were either 'at grade' or had met the objective of a five month gain by the end of the project."

The following conclusion is as true now as it was when written in 1971: "In addition, it appears likely that a similar approach directed to earlier detection of perceptual-motor problems, prior to the development of severe learning lags, has great value for the regular as well as special student."

Mr. President, Our Children Need Vision

Optometrists in vision care are unceasing in their efforts to bring the news to one and all. Conferences, seminars, lectures anywhere and everywhere, locally and worldwide. They give their time as freely to neighbors as they do to influential, top officials. The 1970 report on the White House Conference on Children and Youth, "Vision--Its Place in the World of Children," opened:

"For several decades, the American Optometric Association has enthusiastically taken part in the White House Conference. At the Mid-Century Conference, AOA stressed the effect of the visual process in achievement and personality as well as inter-disciplinary cooperation. At the 1960 Conference, the role of vision in a creative life was our theme.

"AOA would like to see all the professions, agencies and individuals involved in child welfare become fully receptive to the vision care and remedial services offered by optometrists. Optometric services include diagnosing eye health problems, providing developmental vision examinations and therapy, vision therapy, orthoptic and pleoptic therapy, visual aids to the partially sighted (visually handicapped) youngster, visual rehabilitation to the physically and mentally retarded, and acting as consultants to school systems."

It's Never Too Late or Too Early

One of the most exciting aspects of optometric vision therapy is that age is not a deterrent. Under normal circumstances, you're never too young or too old to benefit from this therapy. Some optometrists work with pregnant women, helping them learn to reduce stress in their daily routines and to become aware of the ways in which our habitats and habits influence vision. Around the world, practitioners who offer this therapy have as patients infants and adults in their seventies.

If asked, optometrists everywhere would probably answer as one that the people they most want on their team are parents and educators. These are the individuals who are in the best position to observe the nuances of children's behavior. A pamphlet from the Optometric Extension Program Foundation, "Educator's Guide to Classroom Vision Problems," is par-ticularly useful because of its guide and checklist for adults, parents, school personnel and consulting clinicians.

The material is aimed at helping one to make reliable obser-vations of any aspects of children's visual behavior that might be interfering with academic progress; it stresses that nearly all the visual problems that deter youngsters will not be uncovered by the Snellen Chart or by most stereoscopic devices.

Checklist for Parents & Educators

Appearance of eyes

- one eye turns in or out at any time
- reddened eyes or lids
- eyes tear excessively
- encrusted eyelids
- frequent styes on lids

Complaints when using eyes

- headaches in forehead or temples
- burning or itching after reading or desk work
- nausea or dizziness
- print blurs after reading a short time

Behavioral signs of visual problems

Eye movement abilities

- head turns as reads across page
- loses place often during reading
- needs finger or marker to keep place
- displays short attention span in reading or copying
- too frequently omits words
- writes up or down hill on paper
- rereads or skips lines unknowingly
- orients drawings poorly on page

Eye teaming abilities (binocularity)

- complains of seeing double (diplopia)
- repeats letters within words
- omits letters, numbers or phrases
- misaligns digits in numbers columns
- squints, closes or covers one eye
- tilts head extremely while working at desk
- consistently shows gross postural deviations at desk activities

Eye-hand coordination abilities

- must feel things to assist in interpretation
- eyes not used to "steer" hand movements
- writes crookedly, cannot stay on ruled lines
- uses hand or fingers to keep place on page
- repeatedly confuses left-right directions

The checklist has many other indications listed in two other categories: visual form perception (visual comparison, visual imagery, visualization) and refractive status (nearsightedness, farsightedness, focus problems, etc). All are valuable clues for concerned adults caring for or involved with youngsters.

Scientists Stymied in Quest to Match Human Vision

The *New York Times* reported on September 25, 1984, that "experts pursuing one of man's most audacious dreams--to create machines that think--have stumbled while taking what seemed to be an elementary first step. They have failed to master vision. After two decades of research, they have yet to teach machines the seemingly simple act of being able to recognize everyday objects and to distinguish one from another." The researchers were reportedly scouring the fields of mathematics, physics, biology and psychology for help to achieve the goal of machine vision.

Optometrists would have to agree with these scientists: human vision is not simple. This complexity is one of the main reasons why verification of optometric vision therapy has taken time. "Ten years ago, the only available way to measure eye movements was through observation," explained Dr. Flax in the early 1980s. At that time, the use of exacting instruments and objective evaluation methods enabled researchers like optometrist Harold Solan, clinical professor and Director of the Learning Disabilities Unit at SUNY's College of Optometry, to direct a variety of research, some double blind, aimed at validating optometric vision care. Scientists use infrared optometers to track accommodation and vergence to the nth degree. They are also able to measure binocularity more accurately than ever. By using an electroencephalogram to measure electrical activity in the visual cortex, University of Waterloo vision scientist J. V. Lovosaki, O.D., showed that low plus lenses could strengthen alignment and accommodative stability in some children.

The *Review of Optometry* of May 1985 devoted its lead article to optometric vision therapy, reporting that the National Eye Institute was scheduled to spend $41 million, about a fourth of its budget, on research of the way vision functions. Such research will benefit individuals--and perhaps those puzzled scientists hoping to help computers have vision.

Chapter 8

A Home Guide

Health care today is in a state of transition. We are seeing a positive reorientation embraced by millions, often encouraged by their physicians. The research and work on laughter therapy and the biology of hope initiated by Norman Cousins, the vitamin therapy of Linus Pauling, prayer, biofeedback, balanced nutrition--rather than wait till you are sick and need allopathy, or medical care which treats disease, the emphasis is on holistic health, on homeopathic and naturopathic health care that seeks a state of wellness. Somatic training like Feldenkrais, acupressure work like shiatsu, yoga practice, are valuable preventive practices that are gaining recognition.

Optometric vision therapy is preventive health care much as dentistry is preventive health care. Just as there are times when we need to visit the dentist, so too there are times when we need to visit the practitioner of optometric vision therapy. Often, a program of vision therapy includes procedures to be done at home to supplement office visits. It's preferable to make regular office visits if possible, for several reasons: 1. So that a professional can analyze progress and adjust the workload where necessary. 2. Lens use, a critical factor in this therapy, needs to be monitored for adjustments.

The question of home procedures must always be considered carefully. Some youngsters may need an adult's help, but if the home situation isn't right for that involvement, then it's wise to not use home procedures. In cases, where the patient lives a long way from the practitioner, the patient may be given a home program and office visits will be infrequent. Although it's impossible to duplicate the therapy done in the office, because of lens, prism and equipment use, home programs are of value.

You may already practice self-help. If you are taking the Feldenkrais classes, Awareness Through Movement (ATM), or going to individual practitioners for Feldenkrais, shiatsu or any other types of beneficial body work, you are aware of your needs. Surprisingly, many of our general activities really benefit our vision systems. Just as we're strongly influenced by negative factors such as stress, overwork, poor nutrition and fatigue, so too there are positive factors that may already be part of our daily routine or are simple to add. Relaxation techniques, physical exercise, eye movements, some general, some designed for specific symptoms of vision imbalances such as nearsightedness, are some of the ways to help your vision system, regardless of age or occupation.

Exercise is as valuable for your vision as for your physique and mental awareness. Walking, jogging, jumping rope, weight lifting, aerobics, any and all such programs are good. Yoga is beneficial because it has the additional dimension of deliberate, self-induced relaxation. Yoga also helps you to become attuned to your body's reactions and needs, to develop flexibility both physically and mentally. This is a key point when considering the vision system. If you can be flexible in your body and your mind, you will be able to cope with the demands made on you, whether they are realistic or outrageous. And if your body and mind are flexible, your vision system will be affected in a positive way.

The Value of Regular Visual Relaxation

Perhaps the single most important rule to counter stress and tension in the vision system is regular visual relaxation. It's probably also one of the hardest to learn because it is so simple. It is of great benefit for those who are nearsighted or becoming so. You can literally thwart myopia by relaxing your vision system regularly. These are the steps:

Stop close work every twenty minutes and gaze out of a window or look across the room at a farpoint for a few minutes before returning to your work. The vision system can be relaxed by looking into the distance. You can sit or stand, but be sure that your body is in that state of relaxed awareness one sees in cats. Be aware of the whole room or scene.

Now you don't have to feel guilty about daydreaming because it's an excellent visual habit to learn to take breaks regularly.

Here are vision-relaxing tips borrowed from acupressure techniques. They are similar to yoga practices and the techniques used by massage or shiatsu therapists.

1. Use your thumbs to massage gently under your eyebrows. Start from the inside and slowly work along the eyebrow. Your other fingers can rest on your forehead while you do this.

2. Gently massage the bridge of your nose with thumb and index finger. First press downward then upward.

3. Place your thumbs under your chin, then put your index fingers a finger-width away from nose. Now massage cheeks.

4. Put your thumbs on either side of your forehead, curl your fingers. Use sides of index fingers to massage from the center of the face out, first across the eyebrows, then below the eyes.

If you practice these techniques several times a week, you will feel and look more relaxed.

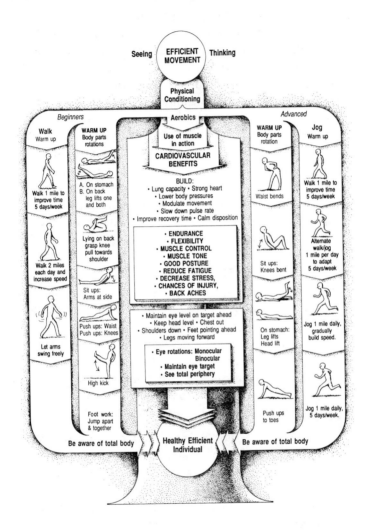

Chart 1. Walking, jogging, aerobics, yoga, Feldenkrais Awareness Through Movement classes, all help to develop and stimulate the efficiency of the vision system so that you work and play to your full potential.

How To Help Your Vision System

The chart on the previous page was developed by Dr. Forkiotis for the Connecticut State Police as part of his program to help the troopers learn how to make their vision systems as efficient as possible. At first glance, the material looks similar to what you might find in any fitness manual. However, if you practice any of these activities regularly, you will enhance visual efficiency and flexibility. In addition to working with the Connecticut State Police, Dr. Forkiotis and several of his colleagues, including Dr. Sol Slobins of Fall River, Massachusetts, and Dr. George Shola of Scituate, Rhode Island, have worked with the Boy Scouts of America, Police Explorer Section, using similar material. The behavioral optometrists screen the young scouts with comprehensive vision analyses and also educate them about good vision habits and the value of caring for the vision system.

Exercises That Benefit Vision

These activities are not new exercises to anyone. For years we've all heard of the virtues of walking and jogging. We've been cautioned to warm up properly and build up to full power carefully. We've learned that when we exercise we do feel better and look better. When vital signs are monitored, improvements can be noted. We build lung capacity and strengthen our hearts. We also recover from excitement more rapidly when we've been exercising regularly.

The points that Dr. Forkiotis adds to the list are an emphasis on total flexibility and an awareness of your vision. How well do you actually use your vision system while exercising? Many people use earphones while they walk or jog and listen to music or self-improvement tapes. Although they may be scanning the area with their eyes while they move, this is not quality use of the vision system. It's preferable to go without the earphones as often as possible and focus on what you see. Move your eyes from side to side, scan the area. Don't let it become a chore, but look carefully at what you see, in a relaxed way. It's also of value to scan as you drive, checking both the road ahead and the side areas just ahead of you.

Concentrate on developing an awareness of what's in your peripheral vision as well as what can be seen ahead of you. Also concentrate on how you move and what difference this makes to the quality of how you see. Remember that a symptom of a vision imbalance such as nearsightedness is found not just in the vision system but actually in the entire body and is shown by the level of total flexibility. When nearsightedness is measured in the vision system, it's actually a measurement of the body's total involvement in this symptom.

Visualization

Athletes improve their performance by visualizing their play before the event. Artists, whether actors, dancers or painters, need to visualize what it is they will be sharing with their audience. When we visualize, we create images and scenes in our mind's eye. Some are better at visualization than others. Once, when visiting Dr. Forrest in New York, this writer spent the evening observing as he guided young doctors of optometry in their residency program for behavioral optometry.

At one point, a request came for Dr. Forrest to step next door to a small room where a young patient had frustrated all of the doctors' efforts to help her. The patient was a shy young girl of nine, whose mother sat patiently with her. Briefly, one of the residents explained to Dr. Forrest that the patient had reported that her eyes were more comfortable with the glasses that had been prescribed by the clinic, but that little or no improvement had been made in her schoolwork. The family and school were concerned over the youngster's lack of reading skills, poor writing and poor spelling. Apparently, no matter how hard the child worked, either at home with an obviously loving, caring mother, or at school, in what the mother said was a good, supportive classroom situation, there was little or no improvement.

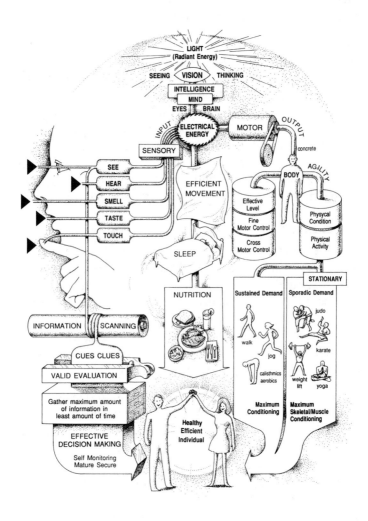

Chart 2. This chart traces the connection between physical activities, physiological reactions and the way the vision system processes information. When we have smooth interaction of all our systems, we work with comfort and efficiency.

Dr. Forrest asked a few questions of mother and child, who grew more and more despondent as they replied, usually in the negative.

"No, tutoring didn't help my reading."

"No, I don't seem able to learn to spell well."

Then, Dr. Forrest introduced a new subject.

"Have you ever tried to see pictures in your mind, has anyone talked to you about doing that?"

"No."

"Let's try now." Dr. Forrest turned slightly so that he was now talking to the residents.

"We're going to try visualization with this youngster."

Then he turned back to face the child.

"You know how to spell your name?"

"Yes.

"Close your eyes and imagine a chalkboard like you have at school. Now on that chalkboard, put the letters of your name."

After a short silence, Dr. Forrest asked the youngster if she was able to do this.

She shook her head.

"That's all right," came the reply. "Open your eyes for a moment. Do you see the chair your mother is sitting on?" The girl nodded.

"I want you to close your eyes and imagine the chair."

Everyone in the room watched intently.

"Do you see the chair in your mind's eye?" The girl nodded.

"Can you put an apple on the chair?"

Nod.

"Now can you move the apple off the chair to the floor?"

Nod.

"That's good," said Dr. Forrest. "Now, I want you to open your eyes while I explain what we're going to do next."

The youngster opened her eyes. She was not smiling but she was pleased with herself.

"Today is Thursday. Can you spell Thursday?" The girl looked at her mother, who nodded reassuringly.

"Yes," came the answer.

"Now, I want you to close your eyes and see the chair again. And I then want you to put the letters of the word Thursday on the chair."

Closing her eyes, the girl concentrated on the task.

"Have you done that?"

"Yes.

"Now, I want you to spell the word out loud, backwards."

This the youngster did, without any difficulty.

When she had finished, she opened her eyes and beamed at her mother.

"That's good. Practice that at home, just for ten minutes or so each day, not too much so that it's tiring and not on days when she's not well. You'll find your spelling and reading will improve," Dr. Forrest said. He turned and left the room. When we were outside in the corridor, he asked me if I had any questions. One came to me.

"Is everyone able to visualize?"

"Not necessarily. Some people can learn, as we just witnessed."

"Do you visualize, Dr. Forrest?"

"No," he answered, after a slight pause. He smiled at me. "I've tried but I am not very successful. Do you visualize?"

"Yes.

"In color?"

"Rarely."

That night, on my way home, I thought about how I'd write about the scene, which I could visualize in my mind almost as well as if I were back in the room.

A Powerful Tool for the Vision System

Visualization is used in optometric vision therapy to improve image memory. This in turn can help in many ways. In the case above, visualization was the way to help a youngster with her spelling and schoolwork. Visualization is also valuable at helping you relax. Imagine one of your favorite places, the beach, the mountains, your garden when the roses are blooming. Put yourself in a comfortable place, doing what you like most--sunning, hiking, gardening--and feel yourself relaxing. In contrast, imagine missing the train, and being late for an important meeting. Feel the adrenalin mounting? Visualization is used in different ways to enhance visual performance.

Check Important Vision Skills

Peripheral vision, as it is used by both eyes simultaneously, in a binocular manner, is one of the most important functions of your visual system. It lets you know where you are. It's also the foundation for the development of size, time and spatial concepts. If you know where you are when walking, balancing or running, you won't stagger or fall. You judge size by this vision skill. Peripheral binocular vision is a vital function of a binocular system. Lack of or inefficient peripheral vision is the major cause of auto accidents. We're not talking about reduced sight or low vision here, but the efficient use of peripheral vision. Check yours by standing in the middle of the room and looking straight ahead. How much of the rest of the room are you aware of? Ask a friend or someone in your family how much they can notice of side areas when they look straight ahead. The following can help you find out the quality of your binocular peripheral vision.

The Brock String Test

This device, three beads or buttons of different colors on a piece of string some three to four feet long, was created by Dr. Frederick Brock, one of the pioneers in the field of optometric vision therapy. It is a good example of the type of simple equipment that can be used to exercise and stimulate the vision system.

When you use the Brock string, you learn a number of things:

- Are you using both eyes as a team all the time?

- Which eye is the "stronger" eye?

- What is the quality of each eye's vision?

- Do you aim both eyes at the same place at the same time?

When you focus on different beads at different times, you can develop valuable eye-teaming skills.

How to Use the Brock String

Thread string through four or five beads and secure them so that they are evenly spaced one from the other. Position the first bead about twelve inches from the end of the string. Attach one end of the string at eye level to a door knob or other convenient handle (or you can hold it yourself), and wind the other end around your fingers. Hold string taut, at arm's length, with the end wrapped around your finger and held against the middle of your nose; look at the bead closest to you. The Brock string can be held still or it can be rotated for focusing and teaming work.

If you're using both eyes together at the same time and aiming accurately at the first bead, it will look as if there are two strings that meet in a V at the bead; the strings seem to go into the beads and come out on the other side, thus they form an X. Each string should be of equal quality, not become fuzzy or indistinct at any place.

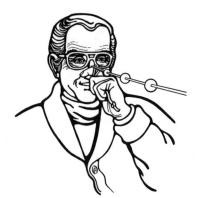

Work with the Brock string may seem simple but the results and benefits of this activity are considerable.

If the strings meet before the bead, you have a tendency to fixate or aim inaccurately, or over-converge. This will cause you to hold your reading material too close--which is stressful. It also might cause you to blur at distance occasionally. If the strings meet behind the button, you are diverging.

If you see two beads side by side, you have difficulty converging. This means you probably hold your reading too far away, causing stress. Lower back problems may also result. If your eyes don't work together as a team, you rarely know it. Where there's a lack of teaming, the individual often uses first one eye then the other. This creates certain behavioral characteristics. You might change your mind a great deal or have difficulty making decisions. Perhaps you have a slow response to a visual activity such as the Brock string. This often indicates a slow starter, maybe even someone accused of being a procrastinator.

Use the Brock string on a daily basis, if possible, if you find your binocularity is not very efficient. Don't overdo it at first if you do have problems, such as the strings meeting in front of or behind the bead at which you aim your eyes. Just as you must gradually build up your endurance for physical exercise, so you must build up endurance for visual exercise. At first, spend about 40 seconds on each bead, preferably at the same time each day, as many times a week as possible. Then, as you improve, you can slowly increase the time you spend on this simple but valuable drill.

You have efficient binocular ability when you see two strings of the same quality. Perhaps you have learned to see the strings in the correct place, but they do not stay visible clearly or steadily but flicker or fade. If so, you need to work consistently at the drill to develop efficient eye teaming that allows you to use both eyes at the same time and see consistently.

It's shocking to realize one doesn't always see consistently. Normally, we're not aware of vision imbalances. It's only when we start using devices like the Brock string that we begin to realize the quality of our perceptions. If you are playing sports--football, tennis, golf, baseball--you may not time your swing at the ball correctly. Analyze your own game. If you see the strings on the Brock string cross behind the bead, you sometimes swing too late. If you see the strings cross in front of the bead, you tend to swing too early.

If our vision systems are not efficient, we need to put far more energy into trying to see accurately than people who have good vision. When you are driving, your brain wants to know where the road is for the left-hand turn. If you cannot see the corner in the road accurately, you will analyze the information over and over in an attempt to understand the visual input. This can be dangerous when you're behind the wheel of a car. In many situations, it can make you seem slow, even stupid.

Test Your Binocular Vision
A simple way to check if you do use both eyes at the same time can be done at home with the cardboard tube from, say, a roll of paper towel.

1. Hold the cardboard tube in one hand, position it in front of one eye and look through the tube.

2. Place your other hand, palm facing you, by the side of the tube, halfway down, at the center of the tube.

3. If you're using both eyes together, you will see a hole in your palm which matches the size of the hole that you see at the end of the tube.

4. If you're not using both eyes together, you will either look down the cardboard tube or just see your hand.

Conclusion

You have binocularity if you see both the tube and the hole in your palm at the same time. You are not truly binocular if you see only one or the other. You probably knew this, if you knew you cannot view 3-D movies. What does this lack of true binocularity mean? It means you do not have accurate depth perception. This imbalance is a drain on energy and leads to stress. It creates difficulties in your perception of your location and the location of objects around you. Walking, driving, sports activities become obstacle courses.

The Benefits of Home Procedures

Often, optometric vision therapy will include procedures to be done at home, if this is practical. The following is included to emphasize the value of home procedures, as part of therapy. This case history involves two family members, mother and son. Each had serious vision difficulties that had gone un-detected despite yearly exams by ophthalmologists and general optometrists.

Mr. and Mrs. Evans, the parents of three boys, knew that their youngest son John, although bright, had much more difficulty learning to read than his two older brothers. John himself would get frustrated at how long it took him to handle his schoolwork at home and in class.

"He was really having a difficult time. It's true to say that even though he tried very hard, he was barely coping with his reading and writing," his parents recall. Now and then, Mrs. Evans had wondered if John's eyes gave him problems. She had noticed even before John started school that at times one eye would turn in a little then snap back, straight again. True, it happened rarely. His mother noticed it when she sat opposite the youngster at mealtimes. One eye would turn in to the nose, just a little, just briefly.

"Probably fatigue, or overexcitement," reasoned Mrs. Evans when she discussed it with her sister. "It's only at special times, birthday parties or big holidays, that I see it happen."

Before John started first grade, his mother took him to an ophthalmologist, who assured her that her son's eyes were fine. Doubt nagged at Mrs. Evans as John so clearly struggled in school. By third grade, she had taken John to several more ophthalmologists. One specialist, who was sure nothing was wrong with John's eyes, said to Mr. and Mrs. Evans, "People make too much fuss over youngsters being slow readers. I know of a lot of boys in medical school who have all their work read to them." Both parents could accept this. When John's homework was read to him, he knew it immediately. If he had to do it by himself, it would take hours and he still didn't have it right. Yet although what the ophthalmologist said seemed reasonable, Mr. and Mrs. Evans were not at all content with the situation. They grew more and more frustrated as they watched their youngest struggle through each day at school. This frustration took them on a constant search for an answer. Surely, they reasoned, eyesight could be a cause, so each year, John's eyes were checked.

By fourth grade, John had been examined by five ophthalmologists. Still nothing was wrong, apparently. One of the specialists had an intriguing theory: a right-handed person whose left eye dominates might have trouble with coordination. When this specialist tested John, he could not find anything wrong with the boy's eyes, but John was left-eyed and right-handed. This could be the source of the problem, theorized the specialist. When Hope Evans questioned this specialist about why one of John's eyes turned in now and then, there was a ready answer.

"One eye is closer to the nose, that's why it seems to you to cross, or turn in occasionally."

The specialist did suggest treatment.

"I've trained an orthoptist," he said. "Someone who works with machines that are used widely in Europe. Telephone her for an appointment. I believe John might have a perceptual problem. If so, she can help."

When Hope Evans took her son to the orthoptist, the use of an opaque patch for John's left eye, the strongest eye, was suggested. The theory was that since the youngster was right-handed, the patch would make his right eye dominant. Hope noticed that the unpatched eye didn't seem to wander the way the left eye had. At dinner that evening, John put his fork in his cheek, instead of his mouth. Patching his strong eye made such a difference to him, he had difficulty finding his mouth!

"Perhaps we're on the right track, at last," Hope Evans said excitedly to her husband. "John certainly isn't managing well with the strong eye covered."

Later, both parents watched in astonishment as John fumbled with the wing of a small model glider he was trying to assemble. Usually, he was quite adept at model-making. This time he could not put the wing in its slot, yet he'd been able to manage this type of work many times before. The wing finally broke as the youngster struggled with it; it was obvious the boy could not see clearly.

At first, John only wore the patch at home and when doing his homework. After a few months, he came downstairs to breakfast wearing the patch on a school day. "I'm going to wear it all day," he announced.

"Even to school?" his mother asked.

"You may have problems with the other children," added his father.

"I'll be finished with the patch much faster."

"How will you feel if the children tease you?"

"I'll tell them I need the patch."

John wore the opaque patch for most of fourth grade. His mother started keeping a careful record of grades for all his work, not just report cards. The boy's marks were regularly in the 80s, a significant improvement. Then, on one of their weekly visits, the orthoptist discovered a serious problem.

"John is losing the sight in his patched eye," she said. "This is something we watch out for, it does happen when an eye is patched for any length of time."

The orthoptist recommended a visit to the ophthalmologist. Technically, John now had nearsightedness in the eye that had been patched. The ophthalmologist confirmed that John had myopia as a result of the patching. Glasses were prescribed. The patching was stopped but the youngster's grades continued to be good and did not slip back to their former, low levels.

At this time, John's mother Hope was working at a nursery school for retarded children. She'd taken the job because she knew it wouldn't involve close work using her eyes, for they were bothering her more and more. She had to keep having the lenses of her glasses changed every few weeks. That Christmas, Hope received a letter from a friend enthusing about a doctor who had treated their retarded child.

Dear Hope,

This doctor is a behavioral optometrist. He worked with Anne [their daughter] for just a few months and the difference is incredible. I've no hesitation in recommending Dr. Edelman to you. He's succeeded with a lot of youngsters where no one else, even specialists like Dr. ---- , has been able to help. I know you've been worried about John's eyes. I thought that in case you still needed help, you might try Dr. Edelman. His office is near you.

At this time, Hope did not contact Dr. Edelman because John seemed to be doing well. A few months after Christmas, however, she decided to call the doctor to discuss Dan, one of the youngsters at the nursery school where she was working. The six-year-old boy had caught her attention because of the way he handled everything he touched, from his lunch to toys. He never looked at whatever was in his hands. He acted as though he were blind, yet Dan had beautiful large brown eyes and could see. Dan was labeled retarded and he still wore diapers. Why doesn't Dan look at what he's touching? Hope wondered. Perhaps the behavioral optometrist could help. She telephoned Dr. Edelman and explained the situation to him.

"What sort of doctor are you?" she asked.

"I'm a doctor of optometry, not an M.D.," was the answer.

"Oh, yes," said Hope. "A dentist is a doctor of dentistry but not an M.D."

"Yes," replied Dr. Edelman. "Bring the child in, I'll examine him."

Hope watched in fascination as Dr. Edelman patiently examined the six-year-old. When the lengthy tests were over, the doctor turned to her and explained what he'd found.

"Dan has never used the center of his eye, the macula."

While the two adults were talking, the youngster sat on the floor, quietly playing with a puzzle, carefully assembling it perfectly, piece by piece. Not once did he look at the puzzle.

"How can they call him retarded?" exclaimed Dr. Edelman. "The child is using his peripheral vision so he doesn't turn his eyes down as you or I would, when we use the center of the eye. He's also developed an unusual ability to use his hands as extensions of his eyes."

"Would you call him legally blind?"

"Not really," replied Dr. Edelman. "With training, I believe he could learn to use his eyes properly. I'd like to talk to his parents about the boy having vision training." (Ultimately, the child had optometric vision therapy and the behavior changes were dramatic.)

"I've never heard about this type of training," Hope said, "although my son has been to quite a few eye specialists."

"The work I do is described as behavioral, developmental or functional optometry. It's called this because the way you perceive your environment influences the way you behave. Optometric vision therapy gives you the opportunity to modify the way you behave because it modifies the way you use your vision system. Not every optometrist practices this therapy. You must take postgraduate courses. The ophthalmologists who saw your son John had specialty training in the diagnosis and treatment of diseases of the eye. That's totally different from treatment of the vision system."

"My eyes have always given me problems," said Hope. "Although I love to sew, my eyes hurt so much when I do close work that lately I tend to avoid it. I've even taken this job at the nursery to avoid close work. Perhaps it would be wise of me to have you examine my eyes."

Within a few weeks, Hope Evans had been examined by Dr. Edelman.

"You do have a vision problem," Dr. Edelman said at the end of the hour-long exam. "To the untrained observer, you seem to use your eyes together. In fact you use your left eye for close work and the other for distance. If you're doing close work, you suppress the input of the eye that's farsighted. When looking in the distance, you suppress the input of the near-sighted eye. Therefore you have monocular not binocular vision, which means you use one eye at a time."

Hope Evans frowned thoughtfully.

"As a child, I had great difficulty with sports. I couldn't catch a ball or play tennis. Yet I could play hockey. Would that have been because of this difference in my eyes?"

"Yes," replied Dr. Edelman. "Tell me, do you get car sick?"

"Violently, I dread long trips by car."

"You probably have severe headaches?"

"Regularly."

"You would find vision therapy a great help," said Dr. Edelman.

Hope Evans started weekly vision therapy with Dr. Edelman. Her program was designed to overcome her particular problems and develop her binocular vision. Most days, she worked at home on procedures also. One involved the use of a red, translucent patch, the other a piece of cardboard.

The Red Patch

Hope happened to be taking therapy with Dr. Edelman in the summer, so she was able to work in good light, which is needed with this procedure. She would cover one eye with the translucent patch and stare around, keeping both eyes open.

If she looked at the white door of her house, at first it would look white, then red. Then, suddenly it would look striped. This meant she was alternating the use of her eyes, not using her eyes together as a team, not fusing the input. She did this for about three weeks, every day for five minutes. After about ten days, when she wore the patch, everything she looked at was pink. Once her system learned to work in this way, she did not lose this ability.

The Cardboard Occluder

Hope used this for four weeks, every day for a few minutes, while she hit a swinging ball. It was designed to help her vision system keep both eyes working together, not one working on distant objects and the other working on near objects. The cardboard, an oblong, about five inches long and two inches wide, was held up in front of one eye, obscuring half the view. Hope would then hit a ball, which was suspended on a string. This procedure was designed to help Hope develop the ability to keep both eyes working at the same time, not shutting off one at far or one at near.

Years later, Hope recalls how insistent she was about doing those procedures regularly at home.

"Once I had learned to do the procedures correctly, I used to worry each day before I started practicing them that I would have lost the ability--but I hadn't. I was desperate to avoid the eye problems that had plagued my family. One of my aunts had serious trouble with her eyes. And a great-grandmother had gone blind at the age of forty. I was frightened because I had already had what I considered was a loss of sight."

A few months after beginning the therapy, Hope had a curious experience. She was out walking on a fine, sunny day. At first, as she admired the sun streaming through the trees, she thought the unusual effect she noticed was just the angle of the sun. Somehow, it reminded her of three-dimensional paintings. Then she realized what she was seeing: the trees in 3-D. The superb effect was stunning to Hope. She'd never seen anything like it. Was this how other people saw the world?

She telephoned Dr. Edelman when she returned home.

"Yes," he confirmed. "You'll gradually have more and more experiences like that. Your 3-D will be patchy at first but it will come."

On her next visit for office therapy, Hope mentioned her son John's nearsightedness, which had been caused by the patching.

"Would you examine him?" she asked.

Dr. Edelman had only one question when he finished John's vision analysis.

"You've been told your son had nothing wrong with his eyes until the nearsightedness developed?"

"Yes, by more than one doctor."

"Come stand behind me and watch. You'll see how his eyes follow this silver ball. Then you'll begin to understand the vision difficulty John's been living with."

Puzzled, Hope Evans walked over and watched as Dr. Edelman slowly moved a small silver ball on a stick from right to left in front of her son. She gasped at what she saw.

"One eye follows the ball smoothly but the other eye jerks back and forth."

"Yes. That's a nystagmoid oscillation. The eye oscillates or moves from side to side."

"What does it mean when both eyes don't move smoothly together?"

"The input to the brain is erratic. This disrupts memory and concentration. When John's reading, he never sees the same information with both eyes. This is terribly confusing for him. He might see the word *READ* with his left eye but the right one is shooting back and forth so rapidly, it will drop part of the word. Maybe the right eye will only catch *RED*, it'll drop the *A*."

"John had a very hard time learning to read. He used to complain, 'Mommy, the page swims in front of me.'"

"Did you ever discuss that with any of the doctors you visited?"

"Yes. The usual answer was, 'He's imagining it, or looking for attention."

"Hardly either. Your son was giving quite a good description of his problem."

"Can you help him?"

"Certainly. You'll have procedures to do at home with John as often as possible, and I'd like to work with him in the office once a week."

Mrs. Evans had to train her visual system so that both eyes worked together all the time at far and near. In this way, she developed binocularity. Her particular problem had not created a learning disability like John's because with only one eye at work, Hope had received consistent input through the vision system.

The input John received through his vision system was erratic. He constantly had to try and mesh two different types of information and try to make sense out of the fluctuations and inconsistencies. John's visual problem was solved when the youngster learned to control his eye movements and move his eyes smoothly together. Then, each eye would send identical input to the brain, where it fused.

Although John had different vision imbalances from his mother, he did use the red, translucent patch and the cardboard occluder. While his mother needed to learn to use both eyes at the same time, not one for near and the other for far, John had to stop shutting off one eye and to use both eyes together and fuse the input. He had been alternating the use of his eyes because of the oscillation, first using one then the other eye, a serious visual habit which leads to learning problems. An important part of the therapy for mother and son was lens use. Each had glasses which they wore for close work and while doing their home procedures. When they were in the office having weekly therapy, Dr. Edelman used a variety of lenses and prisms.

John's mother also found a way to help her son with his homework. She would let him dictate his papers to her and she'd write them. This lasted only a few months, but it proved to be a practical and valuable type of tutoring.

Vision therapy eliminated John's nystagmoid oscillation. The youngster was able to settle down to his schoolwork without the distraction of one eye shooting back and forth and disrupting his memory and concentration. Hope Evans also completed her vision therapy successfully. Mother and son both learned to use their vision systems efficiently. Hope worried about what would happen when the therapy stopped. Would each regress to their old ways? Would any of the problems reappear? She soon discovered that she and John had made permanent changes through the therapy.

Fascinated with behavioral optometry, Mrs. Evans worked in Dr. Edelman's office as an assistant for over fourteen years until her retirement. Today, her son John is a thriving businessman with a fine reputation in his field.

Nutrition, Vitamins and Vision

"Eat your carrots, they're good for your eyes." An international admonition. Is it true? Definitely. Your eyes contain over six million cone cells and 100 million rod cells that convert light into electrical input for your brain. Each of these cells contain 30 million molecules of an important pigment, retinene, that helps them do their job.

Carrots and those leafy greens, like spinach and salad, have large amounts of betacarotene, a nutrient which our bodies convert to vitamin A. The source of all the retinene in your eye's pigments is vitamin A. When you look at objects, those pigments are used up and constantly need replenishment; a process which is increased at night, when a lack of vitamin A may show up as "night blindness." A behavioral optometrist might describe night blindness as slow recovery of vision after flashes of bright light at night. Behavioral optometrists in general are familiar with the influence of nutrition and vitamins on vision. Some have become recognized authorities on the subject, such as Dr. Ben Lane of Lake Hiawatha, New Jersey, Dr. Garry Kappel of Dallas, Oregon, and Dr. Robert Severtson of San Gabriel, California. Dr. Kavner of New York City has also written illuminatingly on this subject in his book *Total Vision*.

Twentieth-century food is often heavily processed and filled with preservatives. All too frequently, the nutrition and vitamin content are not what they were in the days of our grandparents. Couple this lessening of quality and value with an increase in stress and you may well have deficiencies. The eyes are sensitive to even slight deficiencies and as any biochemist will tell you, since we are each enormously individual, the vitamins needed or used by the eyes can vary widely from day to day.

In addition to vitamin A being of specific value for the eyes, vitamins B through E also make necessary contributions to your vision and your welfare. Perhaps a wise first step is to discuss your individual lifestyle, general reactions and health with someone knowledgeable in this field. The growing number of medical practitioners who are turning to homeopathic practice attests that this approach is in growing favor with consumers. Usually, the homeopathic M.D. is conversant with vitamin use, as well as the need for balanced nutrition. Your library probably has a copy of *The Directory of Homeopathic Physicians,* or can locate one by interlibrary loan. Most libraries also have an assortment of reputable books on nutrition and vitamins. While there are many who believe that we get enough vitamins in our food and that supplements are not necessary, enough evidence points to the very real need to take supplements. Partly accelerated lifestyle and stress, partly environmental pollution, partly use of drugs such as birth control pills and antibiotics have combined to increase our need for vitamins.

It was this writer's privilege to edit on the book *Sugar Blues* by William Dufty. This highly recommended book (translated into many languages) urges readers to make their own decisions about what is correct for them--and to think twice about their consumption of sugar, white bread, red meat, caffeine, alcohol, junk food and processed food. Sound advice indeed. As Mr. Dufty notes, if your body is sending you signals in the form of health problems, tune in, don't turn off those signals. Balanced nutrition and vitamin use is definitely accepted as helping many different mental and health problems. Megavitamin or orthomolecular therapy is built around this premise. Physicians who practice orthomolecular therapy, like Dr. Allan Cott of New York, report dramatic results by treating children with autistic problems or learning disabilities with high doses of vitamins. Research proves that megavitamin use helps alcoholism, senility, depression and schizophrenia. You and your vision don't have to have problems to benefit from vitamins and balanced nutrition.

Computer Use

Emily had been employed by the investment bankers, Morgan Stanley, in New York City for five years. The manager of the department, she was responsible for an array of high-tech equipment, from machines to computers. A Skidmore graduate, she thoroughly enjoyed the challenge of meeting the rush demands of the merger and acquisition department. Reports, copies, and memos flooded in chaotically, but when they left, they streamed out in an orderly procession. Emily's department had to be run in two shifts; someone always staffed the department round-the-clock, keeping up with the demand.

After she had selected and supervised the installation of the latest color processing system, a half million dollars worth of equipment, Emily enjoyed using the computer to produce graphs and charts She reached the point where almost half her day was spent on the computer. She also reached the point where her eyes were red and sore and needed eye drops by the end of the day, each day. When headaches started, Emily asked her mother to make an appointment for her to see Dr. Edelman when next she visited Pennsylvania. The family had just learned of the type of vision care he offered, after reading about behavioral optometry in *Suddenly Successful Student*. They had also discovered they lived quite close to the Newtown Square office of coauthor Dr. Edelman. Emily reasoned that although she probably just needed her eyes checked and perhaps some glasses for computer use, she might as well go to someone with Dr. Edelman's credentials.

The appointment was made and Emily and her mother went to the optometrist's offices. Early in the exam, Dr. Edelman asked Emily if anything about her health was bothering her.

"Well, yes," Emily answered. "I know it's not my eyes, but I have been having dizzy spells."

"I believe from my examination that it is your eyes causing this dizziness," Dr. Edelman replied. "But what did you think it might be?"

"I thought I might have a brain tumor," Emily replied hesitantly. Her mother gasped.

"Tell me about the dizzy spells," said Dr. Edelman.

"Well, I can be working at my desk and then get up and be walking across the office and I lose my balance and stagger."

"You don't smoke, do you?"

"No."

"You look very fit, do you work out?"

"Yes, I belong to a health club and go there regularly."

"Yes, your health seems good and from the form you completed, you are in good shape. It's primarily strain from the computer use. You are sitting for long periods at the terminal, creating a new visual distance for your vision system to adapt to. The ciliary muscles go into a spasm, which accounts for the red, strained eyes and headaches. But in addition, you have a tendency to shut down one eye under pressure. At first, when I was examining you I thought I might have to prescribe lenses for day-long use. But your system is so strong and flexible that by the end of my examination I could tell that lenses just for computer use would resolve the situation."

"How does the fact that I'm shutting down one eye make me feel dizzy and stagger?"

"You establish your horizons visually. If you are walking and your brain decides to give one eye, or circuit, a rest, your horizons will change and you will have to adjust to that change. You will stagger while you are making that adjustment."

Emily and her mother exchanged glances of amazement and relief. What they had learned was reassuring, if startling.

"Do I need therapy?" Emily asked.

"No, but you do need the correct lenses to wear for computer use," replied Dr. Edelman.

Once Emily had the prescription filled, she used the glasses for computer work. Within two weeks, the red, sore eyes went away, her headaches stopped and the dizziness disappeared.

That case history sums up the need for the correct lenses as part of the equipment in places where computers are used. Emily had great sight, the traditional 20/20. But she had a natural tendency for one circuit to shut down under pressure. Computer use triggered a high level of this tendency, to the point where she had dizzy spells several times a week. The video display terminal (VDT) of the modern computer is rapidly becoming a common sight in offices, schools and homes. Computer makers find a particularly rich market in school in the United States, where there is a seemingly endless demand for microcomputers. A general estimate has it that by the 1990s, over 35 million people in the United States will be using VDTs. This may be a conservative figure. In the *New York Times* of December 10, 1984, an article on computer use in schools estimated that by 1992, the United States will have 41.3 million public school students, since in 1982 there were 40.8 million such students. The trend is such that a computer for every twenty to fifty students seems a strong possibility.

Many computer or VDT users will have problems similar to Emily's. They may have been able to handle the visual stress of occasional near work but simply will not be able to cope with prolonged nearpoint tasks of the sort that occur with VDT use. Already, the VDT is a "growing source of vision complaints," says the Optometric Extension Program Foundation (OEP). In a comparison between workers using VDTs and those who were not, the users experienced nearly double the incidence of irritated eyes, burning eyes, blurred vision, and fifty percent more eyestrain. Related physical complaints included headaches, aching necks, backs and shoulders.

These symptoms are directly and indirectly related to increased visual stress triggered by the use of VDTS. Visual stress may also be behind the complaints of general body fatigue, reduced efficiency at work, and higher error rates as the day progresses. Behavioral optometrists have found that most of these symptoms are alleviated through a combination of correcting workstation conditions, posture and stress-relieving lenses prescribed for VDT operations. In some cases, vision therapy was recommended to improve visual skills. In one of their pamphlets, "VDTs and Vision, a User's Guide," OEP noted that the "visual care needs of VDT operators differ from those who work with paper and must include detailed analysis of work situations. They listed signs and symptoms of VDT-generated visual stress. Among the direct signs are:

- headache accompanying or following VDT use

- eye strain, or irritated eyes

- blurred vision

- slow refocusing when looking from copy or screen to distant objects

- frequently losing place when moving eyes between copy and screen

- difficulty seeing clearly at distance after prolonged VDT use

- occasional or frequent doubling of vision; changes in color perception

- failure of current lens prescription to relieve symptoms

The pamphlet also listed the following as indirect, visually-related signs and symptoms:

- neck or shoulder tension or pain

- back pain

- excessive physical fatigue when using VDT

- irritability increases when using VDT

- pain in arms, wrists or shoulders when working

- increased nervousness

- lowered visual efficiency and more frequent errors

Suggestions for VDT Workstations

It's possible to help quite a few vision problems by making changes in the working situation. Here are the important points from OEP:

- keyboard, screen and copy are ideally placed when at equal distances from the eyes

- VDT screens should be slightly below eye level (about 20 degrees). Copy should be at the same level as the screen

- locate keyboard so that wrist and lower arm are parallel to the floor

Sometimes, skeptical questions are asked about the accuracy of warnings about computer and VDT use. Executives, who use VDTs rarely, have been known to discount complaints from clerical staff who sit in front of VDTs for much of the work day. Already, the studies point to the very real fact of VDT-induced stress. OEP reported a study by Mourant, Lakshmanan and Chantadisai that found "two hours of VDT usage produced measurable fatigue in the eye accommodation mechanism as well as an increased blink rate." Printed material and VDT images differ in quality. VDT "characters are relatively blurred and have small area flicker. Continuous action of the eye lens may be necessary to achieve proper focus on the relatively blurred characters. The small area flicker also necessitates constant adjustment to varying light levels. Close range viewing of VDTs requires convergence and accommodation of the eyes for sustained periods of time. The ocular muscles controlling eye movements are likely to be exerted beyond their capacity."

In addition to leading to visual stress, Nobel laureate Dr. Roger Sperry says that people react in one or a combination of several ways:

- they avoid doing near work entirely

- they do the work anyway but with lowered understanding and often experiencing discomfort

- they adapt physically in some way, often by becoming nearsighted or by suppressing the vision of one eye

Certainly this tallies with Emily's experience at Morgan Stanley. A leading researcher into the relationship between brain wave production and vision, William Ludlum, O.D., professor of optometry at Pacific University, Forest Grove, Oregon, reports seeing many patients with no previous visual complaints "coming in with VDT complaints. I'm seeing a trend similar to the one which began in the 1960s when fluorescent lighting replaced incandescent lighting in most offices.

"People need to find ways of coping with the additional visual stress.... For normal users with persistent visual complaints, low-plus (stress-relieving) lenses can ease the stress."

In their 1985 publication, "VDTs and Vision," a report on visual problems associated with VDT use and how behavioral optometry can help, OEP reported that: "These visual stress reactions also have been monitored as increases in alpha wave (brain wave) patterns, measured from the visual portion of the brain." These patterns are similar to the signal-to-noise ratio for audiophiles: large scratches on a record are "noisy" enough to interfere with the enjoyment of the music. The alpha wave patterns show significant reductions of signal levels when the person is tested under the same conditions while wearing stress-relieving lenses. These lowered levels are closely associated with learning states--times when a person is able to take in and understand visual information easily.

The Correct Tools for the Work

One of the leading authors of texts and educational material for behavioral optometry, the late Charles B. Margach, M.S., O.D., a professor at Southern California College of Optometry, suggested a concept that has great value for computer users:

Computer work needs terminal spectacles;
they are necessary tools for the job.

In Curriculum II, OEP educational courses, Dr. Margach wrote that "the concept of 'terminal spectacles' is becoming established among VDT users as tools that are required for the job, just as wrenches are viewed as required tools for an auto mechanic." While she was doing so much computer work at Morgan Stanley, Emily definitely needed tools for the job--that is, the correct lenses prescribed for her total vision needs. Since she was under stress from using the VDT and also shutting down one eye as a result of that stress, it was vital that her lenses were prescribed by a behavioral optometrist. Emily is one of the fortunate group who doesn't require lenses when she's not sitting in front of the VDT. For those of us who need to wear glasses or contacts so that we can be visually comfortable with the world around us, if we also work at the computer, the correct lens prescription is even more vital.

Research shows that 30,000 eye movements are required in the course of a day of VDT viewing. For those individuals who are presbyopic (the gradual decline in the ability to focus on near objects, which generally begins to be evident at around the age of forty) or for shortsighted people who wear lenses all the time, tilting the head backward to bring their lenses into the correct position to focus on the line of sight to the VDT screen is very fatiguing. Bifocals or trifocals can be a comfortable and efficient approach for the VDT user when designed appropriately. Dr. Margach suggested these alternatives:

- single vision lenses (not bifocal) focused for a uniform viewing distance of copy, console and screen

- bifocals, located at the proper position for the individual and with the uppers focused for the screen distance and the segments focused for the copy

- half eyes, using the flexibility of frame placement to reduce head movements

As suggested in studies which won the 1981 Nobel Prize for Medicine, visual skills are part of the natural developmental sequence, which begins in infancy. In learning to walk, the child begins by creeping, crawling, standing, walking with assistance, and finally walking unaided. A similar process from gross to fine motor control takes place in the development of vision.

One visual skill builds on another, step-by-step, as the person grows. Many people miss a step, or do not complete a step or must perform visually demanding tasks before an acceptable foundation of visual skills is in place. Visual skills may be developed through optometric vision therapy with its unique lens and prism use. The therapy disrupts inefficient visual habits and helps the individual establish new, more effective visual movement patterns and coordination. The therapy is not designed to build eye muscle strength--the brain controls eye movement, the ocular muscles direct movement. Rather, the purpose of the therapy is to help the patient to develop efficient visual information processing.

Glare and Other Irritations

Behavioral optometrists never weary of reminding patients that glare is fatiguing. When you are working at a VDT, your line of sight is different from ordinary desk work. Usually, the computer screen is raised and this means that overhead light fixtures and large open windows can become irritating sources of glare. Rather than cover a window, it's preferable to reposition the screen or even move the desk or create some changes which will eliminate the glare.

Computer screens may also act as mirrors to reflect images of objects, light sources, even light clothing. Dr. Margach suggested four ways to eliminate reflections:

- move the object

- reduce the object's reflectance

- use an antireflecting screen or filter over the display tube

- tilt the screen either vertically or horizontally so that the reflection is lost

A fifth and surprisingly common way to be rid of reflections is to contort posture a bit. Dr. Margach warned that this is "almost always undesirable because it produces postural and body distortions that soon begin to take their toll."

Finally, a check of your working area is vital. The OEP pamphlet, "VDTs and Vision, A User's Guide," lists these helpful points:

- chairs should provide proper back support and be easily adjustable by the user

- chair height is preferable when feet are flat on the floor and thighs parallel to the floor

- legs and knees should fit under the work table

- screen brightness and contrast should be adjustable by the operator for maximum viewing comfort

- workstation lighting should provide a 10:3 ratio, the screen characters ten times brighter than screen background; room illumination three times brighter than screen background

- each workstation should have an adjustable, shaded copy lamp that can be aimed by the operator without causing screen reflections

- a movable or tiltable terminal is needed to avoid glare and screen reflections

- operators should face into an open space beyond the VDT screen

- clean VDT screens regularly; they attract and accumulate dust

- have focus and image alignment adjusted frequently to reduce visual stress

- take a short, regular break; demanding VDT workloads benefit from a short change from VDT work each hour

The cardinal rule in behavioral optometry is to relax the vision system every twenty minutes by staring into the distance. This is not easy to remember but you will make fewer errors and be able to work for long stretches without discomfort if you have routine breaks.

How To Help Your Child's Vision

Most babies are born with healthy eyes, free from disease and vision problems. Generally, their entire vision system is in good shape. Over those early years, the impact of the environment and lifestyle affects the vision system just as much as health does. The critical first stages in the newborn's development, however, are dependent on how well the child learns to use the vision system. Since infants spend a large part of their time learning to see, parents of newborns will be delighted to read there's a great deal they can do to help infants develop healthy, balanced vision systems.

Simple, effective ways to help come from the American

Optometric Association's background paper on infant's vision and the guidelines developed over the years by the Infant's Vision Clinic at the State University of New York's College of Optometry in New York City (formerly under the direction of Dr. Elliott Forrest). Bright wallpaper, moving the crib now and then, a colorful mobile, feeding your baby from different sides--this type of variety and movement will encourage and stimulate balanced vision development.

Early Visual Stimulation

Keep a dim light burning in the nursery at night so the infant will be able to look around and see the room when awake. Move the crib regularly, as well as the baby's position in the crib to allow the child to respond to light from different directions. Use clear bumper guards if possible so vision is not obstructed.

Approach, change, feed and play with baby from different positions. Talk to your child as you move around the room, so the infant has a moving object to follow. During the day, place the child in different rooms so that new sights, objects, patterns and different light will stimulate the vision system.

For the first two months, keep a bright mobile dangling outside the crib to provide variety and movement. At about eight weeks, move the mobile over the crib so baby can touch it. This permits reinforcement of tactual and visual information.

Keep reach-and-touch objects within baby's focus, about eight to twelve inches. Objects should be large enough to prevent baby from swallowing them.

You can have more than one interesting object such as the mobile for baby to observe but don't go overboard. Printed sheets and an abundance of toys hanging above and on the side of the crib can overwhelm an infant and actually slow development. Moderation is the key.

Dangle a toy or rattle a few inches above your baby and slowly move it up and down or around to encourage the development of eye tracking skills.

Carry your child in an upright position against your shoulder so that the baby has a range of visual stimulation.

Help the two- or three-month-old hold and shake a rattle.

Switch hands.

Play peek-a-boo by holding the baby's hands in front of her or his face.

Provide blocks, rattle, balls and other toys for baby to touch, bang and throw. Use objects large enough so they can't be swallowed. As the child gets older, make available toys, including pots and pans, to stack, nest, build, string, toss, push, pull, pound, take apart and put together.

Avoid using a play pen or crib for hours on end. When eventually your child is crawling, this is an activity that helps eye-hand-foot coordination. Crawling also offers the child the chance to explore spatial relationships. Early walkers who miss the opportunity to crawl may not learn to use their two eyes together as adequately as babies who spend a great deal of time crawling. Allow your child the freedom to crawl and explore in a safe environment.

Talk to your child, explaining what you are doing in adult language.

Provide floating bath toys.

You may be surprised (and even a trifle sorry) to hear that letting your baby repeatedly drop toys from the highchair (which means you get to pick them up ad nauseam) develops eye-hand coordination skills and the spatial information needed to release and throw objects. Now you know how important this is, perhaps it won't seem such a maddening task!

From eight to twelve months of age, babies are starting to walk, talk, take things apart and put them together again. They can now judge distances fairly well, can throw things with precision, and are ready to begin handling smaller items. At this stage of vision development, you can do the following to help:

Name objects when talking to your baby to encourage associating words with what is seen. This also helps in vocabulary development.

Provide books of sturdy cardboard so your child can learn to manipulate the pages.

Give your child toys or household objects to take apart and put together again, such as snap-lock beads, blocks, stacking and nesting toys or plastic measuring cups and spoons.

When you provide small objects for your baby to handle (but not so small that they can be swallowed), you are introducing the child to the first step in learning the hand-eye coordination skills needed for drawing and writing.

Between one and two, a child's eye-hand coordination and depth perception should become well developed. Now is the time for parents to help youngsters refine and further develop vision skills. Helpful activities include the following:

Roll a ball back and forth to your child. This helps him or her learn to follow an object with the eyes.

Provide building blocks, balls of all shapes and sizes, even a zipper. Playing with small objects will help improve coordination of fine motor skills and small muscle development.

Let your child ride a rocking horse or four-wheeled toys and wagons that can be straddled and pushed with the feet. This will help increase eye-hand-foot coordination. Two-year-olds are highly interested in exploring their environment and in looking and listening. They are beginning to speak in sentences and enjoy using pencils, markers or crayons.

Now you can begin to prepare your child to visualize by reading or telling stories; these activities will also help in the preparation for learning to read.

Allow plenty of time for activities outdoors.

Provide drawing and writing materials which develop an awareness of boundaries and also develop visually directed hand movements.

Beanbag or ring toss games, toys that have pegs to be hammered, toys that need to be sorted by shapes and sizes, puzzles, building blocks--all are good for this age group.

Toys, Games & Your Child's Vision

The American Optometric Association has published a helpful pamphlet on this subject, with the assistance of Dr. Joel Zaba, who has a great deal of experience with youngsters. Dr. Zaba comments that "most of the time your child is at play, the eyes are a part of the action. You can find a lot of ways to use playtime activities, games and toys to help your child, regardless of age, learn or sharpen many different vision skills. And it can be done without interfering with the carefree fun and joy of playtime.

"Inexpensive homemade toys and simple childhood games can be just as effective as purchased toys. When buying toys, select those that are well made and appropriate to the child's age and maturity level. Manufacturers often give suggested ages for a toy but keep the individual child in mind because children develop at different rates, a key factor in knowing and nurturing vision.

"Buy the proper eye safety equipment for older children and be certain they wear it when participating in sports hazardous to the eyes and when using chemistry sets, shop tools, BB guns or other items with the potential to cause eye injuries. Most eye injuries suffered by children occur during play or sports activities and can be prevented.

"The following list of toys and activities for infants from birth through five months will help stimulate your baby's sense of sight.

"Those suggested for older age groups will help develop or sharpen your child's general eye movement skills; eye-hand coordination skills necessary for writing and sports; shape and size discrimination skills needed for reading; and visualization and visual memory skills needed for comprehension and for the ability to visualize in the abstract."

Birth through 5 months Toys: Sturdy crib mobiles and gyms, bright large rattles, rubber squeak toys. Activities: Peek-a-boo, patty-cake.

6-8 months Toys: Stuffed animals, floating bath toys. Activities: Hide-and-seek with toys.

9-12 months Toys: Sturdy cardboard books, take-apart toys, snap-lock beads blocks, stacking/nesting toys. Activities: Roll a ball back and forth.

One-year-olds Toys: Bright balls, blocks, zippers, rocking horse, riding toys pushed with the feet. Activities: Throwing a ball.

Two-year-olds Toys: pencils, markers, crayons, bean bag/ring toss games, peg-hammering toys, sorting shapes/sizes toys, puzzles, blocks. Activities: Read to child, outdoor play, catch.

Three- to six-year-olds Toys: Building toys with large snap-together parts, bead stringing, puzzles, finger paint, modeling clay, simple sewing cards, tricycle, sticker book/games. Activities: Climbing, running, balance beam, playground equipment.

7 years and up Toys: Bicycle, jump ropes, pogo sticks, roller skates, different size and shape balls, target games, more sophisticated building toys, puzzles, remote-control toys, timed shape/size sorting games, tossing between players activities. Activities: Cycling.

The list above is far from complete; it is intended as a basic collection. You can aid your child's visual development in many other ways. Use your creativity and consult your optometrist for suggestions on specific toys and activities.

The Vision Exam

For decades now, parents have been counseled by the various organizations such as the Gesell Institute for Human Development, the American Optometric Association and the College of Optometrists in Vision Development to make an appointment with a behavioral (functional or developmental) optometrist before a child's third birthday for that first, thorough vision exam. After that, unless obvious problems develop, annual optometric exams are recommended.

Research has highlighted the need for an exam even earlier, within the first four to six months of life. A May 1985 article in the *Review of Optometry* quotes scientists and behavioral optometrists around the country agreeing that "clinicians have a better chance of shaping the visual system when they can catch problems early."

Scientists now know that animals go through a crucial period during the early months, a formative time for the visual cortex. "Cross-circuiting cell development during this critical time can destroy the ability to see binocularly, and impair acuity and contrast sensitivity." Neurophysiologist Steven Cool of Pacific University School of Optometry, who is producing definitive research in support of behavioral optometry, says that some of the techniques of optometric vision therapy, such as yoked prisms, actually "pry open a 'sensitivity gate' to that critical period" which may not be as critical in humans as in animals.

"In the first year of life, the human visual system develops at a very rapid rate," says Terry Hickey, director of vision research at the University of Alabama. "During this period, it's essential that the visual environment appear absolutely normal. The two eyes should work in concert, and anything that distorts vision should be corrected." For that reason, behavioral optometrists are encouraging parents to bring their infants in for a comprehensive vision exam during the first few months of life.

"We need to identify deficits or defects" that can affect binocularity in the first few months, says Dr. Jack Richman, a professor at the New England College of Optometry. Tests for infants are not complicated and surprising though it may seem, it is possible to practice optometric vision therapy on small babies.

How Long Does The Exam Last?

A thorough optometric exam of a youngster takes from thirty to sixty minutes on the first visit and includes a variety of tests. While these tests may vary with individual needs, exams should cover:

- a review of the family's health history; facts about the child's birth, development and health

- examination of the eye's exterior and interior for signs of disease or general health problems such as diabetes, that may show up in the eyes

- tests of the child's current ability to see sharply and clearly at near and far distances (this includes tests for amblyopia)

- tests to determine near- and farsightedness and astigmatism

- a check of eye coordination and eye muscle function to be certain the eyes work together as a team

- a test of the ability to change focus easily from near to far and vice versa

- a check for any indications of crossed eyes or indications that the child is not using one eye

- a test of depth perception

- motor tests to check eye-hand-foot coordination

- a test to determine the child's dominant eye

Preschoolers

These youngsters need active play to develop eye-hand-foot-body coordination skills but they also need to stimulate development of fine motor skills and the vision skills necessary to learn to read. Be sure to allow your youngster plenty of time for:

- climbing, walking a balance beam and enjoying playground equipment

- looking at picture books, sometimes with you, too

- using a stand-up chalkboard for drawing and early writing skills; painting with finger paints; Some children are capable of playing when given the appropriate material, others need to be shown and encouraged

- time with you, but time also alone and with other youngsters

Symptoms of Vision Imbalances

Preschoolers may signal problems with their vision in a variety of ways. These include staring into space; holding the body rigid when looking at a distance; scrunching up the face when a visual task is involved; covering or closing one eye; consistently sitting close to the television set; holding books closer than six inches from their eyes; irritability; signs of hyperactivity; avoidance of looking at books or television; lack of organization in play; short attention span for child's age.

If this type of behavior occurs, a thorough optometric exam that includes vision development tests is valuable. An exam that only checks the child's ability to see clearly (20/20 sight) will not uncover difficulties in the development of the child's vision skills.

Be watchful during school years

Academic and social pressures may have drastic effects on

the vision system of our youngsters. Yet these changes may be so gradual that most children are not aware of them. If they are tested at school, they can often pass the eye chart test. Don't be deceived by 20/20 sight, it is merely one aspect of the vision system's functioning. Be aware of more than twenty other visual skills that are vital to learning, behavior and health. Early diagnosis and treatment can help to prevent, correct or slow down vision imbalances that will otherwise interfere with a child's learning, recreation and self-image.

Time is Needed for Maturity

Your infant is barraged with visual stimuli from birth. As babies mature, they begin to fix their vision on objects and forms. This is the beginning of the development of perception. Gradually, the differences in various objects are discerned. If we can't perceive differences, the relationship of objects and activities will be the same and our experience will be lacking or inappropriate. If this happens, perception is either poor or inadequate or inaccurate.

Chronological & Developmental Ages Differ

Just as our individual rates of progress vary, so too there is a difference in the rate at which vision systems and bodies mature. Coupled with this is the difficulty in measuring the success of any therapy because of the differences in individuals and situations. Just as one individual will need to wear braces until the orthodontist can measure an appropriate improvement, so must the optometrist who practices vision therapy evaluate each situation on its own merits.

Dr. Richard Apell likes to tell about the results of treatment for a patient who had long shown the type of behavior and poor academic performance associated with vision dysfunction. When finally the young woman decided to come for vision therapy, the analysis showed a vision imbalance which was definitely triggering the school problems and erratic behavior. Yet to the astonishment of the behavioral optometrist at Gesell, the expected changes and improvements did not materialize, despite the vision therapy. The lack of progress was discussed with the other Gesell departments and further testing done. The results from the nutritional evaluation showed a low thyroid. When this was brought into balance, the vision therapy began to have an effect and the changes were marked.

"If we hadn't treated the individual as a whole, the optometric vision therapy would not have had much of a chance," say Dr. Apell. "Emotional difficulties, physical factors, nutritional imbalances, family pressures or problems at home can all contribute to stress which in turn has a disastrous effect on the vision system."

The Vision System's Development

From birth to eight weeks, the infant is monocular, uses one eye at a time. That's why you need not worry if now and then you see one eye turn in or out. Your baby needs time to learn to use all aspects of its vision system. At approximately two months, infants begin to develop control over binocularity, or the simultaneous use of both eyes. They are able to converge their eyes and often show the ability to see both near and distance objects.

By four months, there is a general awareness of the world around them. At five months, the eye-head control is much stronger and the ability to examine objects at near range grows. In the six month there is usually some teaming of eye-hand responses. This grows in the following months so that the child starts to develop motor coordination and can look around and observe activities.

By ten months, the infant is treating the world as a whole, unified situation. Creeping begins around now, coupled with rising to hands and knees. A reduction in visual attention often occurs as the child begins to develop and use balance and visual-motor relationships. Often, by the time babies are a year old, they begin to walk and all their attention has to go into developing balance and coordination. It is typical at this age to find slightly less of the visual ability that was shown a month or so ago. As balance improves, visual attention will also grow.

Over the next twelve months, one can watch as the infant develops stronger and stronger visual abilities, looking actively and carefully at its surroundings and becoming more and more sure of eye-hand coordination. At approximately thirty months, the child will become easily distractible because of the high use of peripheral vision. By the age of three, a child is usually able to plan in advance, and pays attention to eye-hand coordination. Now the vision system is more central so that concentration develops--the youngster will draw rather than scribble.

At about three and a half, the child will seem to be less confident and question abilities. Often, there is a fear of high places. By the age of four children usually understand symmetry. They become quite assertive and show the ability to shift their attention comfortably. The five-year-old is able to match according to size and shape and will usually choose to deal with one thing at a time. Their ability to make vertical strokes is stronger than their ability to make horizontal strokes. At six a child may appear clumsy and unsure and the behavior may be erratic. By seven, a child will often start to print in smaller letters. They may be withdrawn and easily frustrated.

By the age of eight, many youngsters become quite expansive and their social behavior is good. Writing becomes more balanced and uniform, and often children are comfortable at shifting activities. The nine-year-old shows increasing self-awareness and motivation. Their sense of responsibility and ability to focus their attention is good. By the age of ten, this sharp focusing is somewhat reduced and the balance between their self-awareness and their interaction with the world becomes more even.

We May Need a Baker's Dozen

Usually, our vision systems take an average of twelve years to mature. Individual rates of growth, development and progress vary. Physical and psychological factors affect the vision system and what causes distress to one person will have little or no effect on another. The Gesell Institute has always urged that a child's chronological age not be used to determine grade placement. It's preferable to consider other factors; one of the most important is vision.

Chapter 9

Help Is Here

Practitioners of optometric vision therapy are spread across America. They are also to be found in thirty-five other countries, including Australia, Belgium, Denmark, France, Italy, Japan, the Netherlands, the Scandinavian countries, Spain, and Switzerland. Many of the fifteen colleges of optometry in the United States have clinics like the Eye Institute at the Pennsylvania College of Optometry.

The Eye Institute has been open since 1978, and Dr. Mitchell Scheiman, Chief of Pediatric and Binocular Vision Service at the Institute, guides a facility which sees some 2,500 new patients a year. They provide vision therapy to some 100 patients a week, or 5,000 visits a year. Connecticut's renowned Gesell Institute of Human Development, which had offered postdoctoral training in behavioral optometry from the 1950s until it closed in 1990, saw approximately 2,300 cases for therapy annually at its clinic.

Finding A Practitioner

The traditional ways we all have used to find a good practitioner in any field are just as appropriate for behavioral
optometry. Referral sources include teachers, guidance counselors, psychologists, educational centers and word-of-mouth
recommendations from satisfied patients. When you set out to
find a behavioral (functional or developmental) optometrist in
your area, the most direct source might well be your local
general optometrist. Not all optometrists know of or understand the specialty of behavioral optometry, however, so you
can't always expect guidance from these practitioners. You do
have other professional sources, fortunately. You can contact
either the College of Optometrists in Vision Development, the
Optometric Extension Program Foundation, the colleges of
optometry, or even any of the practitioners mentioned in the
book, if you are fortunate enough to live in their area. For
addresses, see the section in this chapter, Professional Organizations, and the list of colleges in the backmatter.

Always Ask For The Therapy By Name

If you have a youngster or an adult in the family who has
learning, health or behavior problems and hasn't yet had a
behavioral optometric vision exam, why not have one done
promptly? It might well reveal vision imbalances that have
been missed by conventional optometric and ophthalmological
examinations and which could be corrected with the proper
treatment. Don't hesitate to phone to discuss your needs.
Remember to ask clearly for a practitioner of optometric vision
therapy.

Ask how long an exam usually takes. You cannot have a
thorough behavioral vision exam in less than thirty minutes;
often it takes a minimum of forty-five to sixty minutes. This
does not include the use of eye drops, of course; in fact, it is
wise to have your vision system checked without the use of
drugs; their use is appropriate at other times. Remember that
there are a basic twenty-one points of your vision system to be
checked. At the Gesell Institute, frequently a visual analysis

lasted up to ninety minutes. This was because many of their patients had severe learning problems and more than thirty visual skills that are important to learning were tested.

When you have been given the name of a practitioner, make sure you receive "yes" answers to each of the following questions, which are from pamphlets published by the Optometric Extension Program Foundation:

- do you make a full series of nearpoint vision tests?

- do you make work- or school-related visual perception tests?

- do you provide full vision care including visual training in your office, or will you refer me to a colleague if needed?

- will you see me again during the year, and periodically, to determine my progress?

One Student's Search

The furious pace of a nuclear civilization has disrupted the harmony of our vision systems, which were well suited for the farmer, hunter or sailor of earlier times. The close work, miniaturization and pressured situations of twentieth-century life conspire to create vision imbalances. In turn, these imbalances force us to adapt in a myriad ways, some subtle, others not so subtle. Graduate students in particular have an overwhelming amount of close work to handle. Many find the reading and studying difficult, but are not aware that the difficulty lies in their vision systems. Andrew Barnston is a second-year medical student--for the second time. Until he was referred to Dr. Forkiotis, he had struggled desperately with unresolved but chronic health problems. Ultimately, he had been sent for psychiatric counseling; he had to rely on medication to help with the severe headaches, pain, numbness, dizziness, anxiety, panic attacks and mental confusion.

Fortunately for Andrew, when he was home for the Christmas

holidays in 1987, his parents urged him to consult Dr. Forkiotis, about whom they had heard wonderful reports.

"What's the point of going to this doctor when I have to return to college in a few weeks? I'm hundreds of miles away. I can't possible go to him for therapy," Andrew protested.

"From what we've heard, it's a combination of lenses and therapy. Why not at least find out if the glasses you are wearing are correct? If therapy is suggested, perhaps Dr. Forkiotis can recommend someone," replied his father.

"I'm on Ativan, three or four times a day, and I've been seeing the psychiatrist regularly. All the other practitioners couldn't find anything, from the neurologist to an ophthalmologist. Why would an optometrist help?"

"Andy, you told us before dinner you've been in constant pain. I know you've been to a lot of different people. Perhaps you haven't found the answer, yet. How could it hurt to go to one more doctor?" his mother asked gently.

At the optometrist's office, Andy was astonished when halfway through the vision exam, Dr. Forkiotis said, "Looks as though you made the right decision to come here, I definitely find causes why you are having some of your difficulties. Unless I'm sadly mistaken, different lenses will help substantially with the type of health problems you are experiencing."

Later, as Dr. Forkiotis looked over the list of Andy's problems, he shook his head.

"If practitioners would make sure that patients with problems like these have a behavioral vision exam, you would have been helped earlier."

Andy's list read:

- increased awareness of floaters in both eyes

- gastrointestinal pain and nausea

- "dots" that seem to move about randomly and very rapidly, especially if looking at blank wall or open sky

- dizziness

- panic attacks

- weight gain

- increased awareness of afterimages, especially halos around people's heads

- photophobia [morbid dislike of light]

- choking or suffocating feelings during panic attacks

- feelings of anxiety, fear of dying, confusion

- filmlike substance passing in front of eyes if looking from side to side

Although Andy could see clearly, his eyes hurt when he wore the glasses prescribed for him by the practitioner he had visited before going to Dr. Forkiotis. This was because the lens prescription was inaccurate for Andy's vision needs. The visual exam by Dr. Forkiotis revealed a high degree of exophoria (a tendency for the eyes to turn out), both at near and far. The exophoria was only visible through the special optometric tests.

A vision imbalance such as this has been known to trigger the type of symptoms from which Andy was suffering. When Dr. Forkiotis put a certain prism in front of Andy's eyes, the young man's perception of the office changed radically and immediately. He literally felt stable, not dizzy, confused or panicky. His breathing slowed and deepened. Dr. Forkiotis prescribed two sets of lenses, one pair of bifocals, the other set to be used for close work.

Andy's new glasses arrived before he had to return to college. He wore them and found that the various painful and disorienting symptoms suffered over the past months were greatly reduced. His fiance, a physician in obstetrics-gynecology remarked on his calm attitude and also noticed that he held his body differently, particularly when he was driving. Andy's family also noticed a more relaxed attitude.

Dr. Forkiotis also prescribed nasal occluders for Andy to use if he was under severe stress. Nasal tapes, as the occluders are generally called, provide valuable therapy since you do not necessarily have to visit the office to benefit from the procedure. The occluders expand your visual field and make you become more peripherally aware. Some people, especially those who are nearsighted, find the occluders very relaxing. It's also disruptive therapy, since it breaks up the habitual way you have of using your vision.

Strips of tape, in Andy's case translucent scotch tape, are placed on the inner half of each lens. Nasal occluders are very effective in changing visual habits, and since they are used with the correct lens for your particular vision needs, they are highly individual, a truly custom therapy.

A week after Andy had returned to college, Dr. Forkiotis received a phone call from him.

"Doctor, I've had such a good week, despite working hard, but that's not all. When I went to my psychiatrist and explained how you'd helped me, he told me he knew about behavioral optometry and had only the highest recommendation for it. He told me both his children had been in optometric vision therapy and were helped greatly. 'If you have been told by a behavioral optometrist that vision imbalances were triggering your difficulties, then it's possible that you can stop your visits to me,' he said. He also suggested that we begin tapering off the medication." Andy laughed.

"You know what else he said? That I be very careful to follow your instructions to the letter."

A few weeks later, Dr. Forkiotis received a letter from Andy.

Dear Doctor,

I truly enjoyed learning from you during my short visit at home. You "opened my eyes" to many areas of vision physiology and its relationship to the entire body.

I feel very strongly that part of my lack of success at my first attempt at medical school two years ago was indeed due to my not being diagnosed as a visual problem with severe degree of exophoria. The past year for me has been sheer hell. Headaches, visual problems, anxiety, panic attacks, weight gain, confusion at times, dizziness, and gastrointestinal upset.

All the physicians ruled out organic causes and I was ultimately referred to a psychiatrist. You are one of the most compassionate, intelligent, and "humane" physicians I have ever met and I thank you for all that you have done for me. You can rest assured that I will spread the word of behavioral optometry to my fellow classmates, professors and future patients.

How to Evaluate Health Care

Andy had been seen by several different physicians, general practitioners. He was placed on eight weeks of medication, three times daily. When he had finished the medication, Andy still suffered from the various symptoms. He was then referred to an otorhinolaryngologist in an attempt to find the cause of his pain and dizziness. After several visits to this specialist, he was given different medication to use as needed and sent home.

Andy then visited an ophthalmologist, who diagnosed an acute inflammation of the iris and prescribed daily use of a solution that kept Andy's right eye dilated for over four weeks. This was a particularly painful episode for Andy and at the end of it, his situation had improved little. The next step was a visit to a neurophthalmologist who disagreed with the previous diagnosis. A new prescription was given Andy for distance eye glasses, and he was advised to return if problems occurred.

Several weeks later, Andy's old symptoms returned in full blast. This time, Andy went to the clinic at his medical school, which is a teaching hospital. A Cat scan of the skull was ordered but Andy was allergic to the dye and the Cat scan was canceled. His hearing was tested and found to be good. Next, Andy was sent to a neurologist and more tests were ordered. Medication was prescribed in an attempt to ease his pain. Finally, the clinic suggested that Andy see a psychiatrist since a neurosis was suspected. Psychotherapy was begun and Andy was placed on a tranquillizer to be taken three or four times a day to control his anxiety. The diagnosis was that Andy had a panic disorder.

It would seem from the results of Andy's visit to Dr. Forkiotis that the various diagnoses were not accurate and the medications were not appropriate. Dr. Forkiotis was able to reduce Andy's painful symptoms within a few days by prescribing the correct lenses for Andy's vision needs.

A useful book published by Simon & Schuster in 1988, *Playing God: The New World of Medical Choices,* by Dr. Thomas Scully and Celia Scully, discusses the warning signals to alert you to the fact that you may not be receiving proper health care. Dr. Scully also includes an in-depth look at the patient's Bill of Rights, when to blow the whistle on your doctor, nurse, hospital or clinic and how to do it effectively. To this, we add our "classic cliches." Be wary if a health care practitioner comments, "There's nothing wrong." When you are sitting in the physician's office in pain, or have endured pain in recent days, clearly something is wrong. When one exam doesn't find a cause for your difficulties, a more accurate answer would be, "I don't know what's causing your problem, but I will refer you to...." Be particularly wary of the comment, "It's psychological," if a referral to psychotherapy isn't made.

Health care is at the best of times a complex blend. An informed consumer learns about available options. Always remember the ground rules to safeguard yourself: tests are necessary and invaluable if you are trying to discover what ails you, but before you embark on the exotic and expensive variety, once you've covered the preliminary, basic tests, consider the wisdom of having a comprehensive vision analysis by a qualified practitioner of behavioral optometry. When Allan Cott, M.D., advises that any physical examination which does not include a complete vision analysis is an incomplete examination, he is drawing on years of experience as a practicing physician.

College Clinics

Many of America's fifteen colleges of optometry have clinics that offer various types of vision care. Most also have faculty who practice behavioral optometry privately. Be sure to ask for behavioral, developmental or functional optometric vision care. The organizations mentioned later (addresses are also given), usually have directories of practitioners. Call or write these groups and they will send you details on optometrists in your area who offer optometric vision therapy.

A number of centers around the country offer behavioral optometric and psychoeducational diagnoses and therapy geared either to slow learners or the learning disabled. Again, an excellent reference source is one of the professional organizations. If you have difficulty finding addresses for clinics, centers or practitioners, one of the professional groups whose names and addresses follow may be able to help but doublecheck that practitioners actually practice behavioral optometry by asking questions like those mentioned in the section "Finding a practitioner," at the beginning of this chapter. If you are comfortable doing so, it's a good idea to ask for a patient's name as a reference.

Insurance Pays

In a May 29, 1985 article in the *Wall Street Journal*, it was reported that a spokesperson for Aetna Life & Casualty Company said Aetna has offered coverage for optometric vision therapy for "at least a decade." Aetna was also quoted as saying "we're convinced of its value."

It is not surprising to find that medical insurance coverage for optometric vision therapy varies from state to state and from company to company. Simple but sound advice comes from the optometric consultant to Blue Cross-Blue Shield of Greater New York, Dr. Irwin Suchoff: Read your policy.

Look for exclusions in your policy. If optometric vision therapy is not specifically excluded, then it must be paid for.

However, if optometric vision therapy is included, often the insurance company has the choice of deciding which health care professional you visit. So this is the next fact to establish:

Is your coverage for optometric or ophthalmological care?

In the majority of states, insurance guarantees "Freedom of Choice." Yet again, the interpretation is open to different perspectives. Despite the so-called Freedom of Choice, the insurance company may be able to decide your choice. The final authority rests in the insurance laws in each individual state. If your policy is with an insurance carrier and not the company, the carrier does not always have to abide by insurance law.

An excellent publication, "Vision Therapy and Insurance: A Position Statement," was published in 1986 by the State University of New York State College of Optometry. The editor was Dr. Nathan Flax. It's possible that your local behavioral optometrist will have a copy of this helpful material. It's useful to know that in the past there's been confusion over the codes developed by the American Optometric Association, which differ from the medical codes.

COIT is the code for diagnosis by optometrists

COPT is the code for treatment by optometrists

> *In March 1980, that remarkable arbiter of consumer welfare, Ralph Nader, told a symposium of health care professionals that his findings supported the fact that optometric vision therapy is effective.*

Visionary Vistas

American optometrists who practice optometric vision therapy are dedicated to sharing this health care with practitioners in other countries. To do this they must venture far afield. Dr. Greg Gilman of Quincy, California, has literally traveled around the world lecturing on behavioral optometry. The trip took place in 1983 and 1984 and Dr. Gilman had the route and his seminars planned eighteen months before he left. He and his wife traveled continuously for eighteen months and visited fifty countries.

"An average of seventy-five people attended each seminar, although one seminar attracted 2,500 optometrists," says Dr. Gilman. "In Zaire, forty percent of all the optometrists in the country attended. That's two, because although the population of Zaire is 25 million, they only have five optometrists."

Already, he has stimulated students and practitioners to visit America and learn more about behavioral optometry. Among the countries he visited were those of northern Europe. Dr. Gilman reported that behavioral optometry seemed to be heading in new directions in the Scandinavian nations, Belgium and the Netherlands. In 1985, two young Belgium optometrists founded a school to teach behavioral optometry. One of the school's founders visited behavioral optometrists in New Jersey and began a visual training practice on his return to Belgium.

The Optometric Extension Program Foundation study group in the Netherlands organized several seminars for Dr. Gilman. One was attended by seventy-five physicians, another by eighty people in specialties which use sensory integration theory, and a third drew 220 teachers for an all-day seminar. Those Dutch optometrists who practice optometric vision therapy refer to themselves as "optologists" to distinguish themselves from their colleagues who practice general optometry.

Now back in practice in Quincy, Dr. Gilman has published a book about his world trip. He feels that at least half of it is understandable to the general reader. The book, *Behavioral Optometry,* has the type of material that Dr. Gilman used for his seminars, as well as general information about behavioral optometry. At a cost of $30 (plus $3 shipping and handling), this is a valuable addition to libraries personal and public. Dr. Gilman's book can be ordered from OEP's Vision-Extension, Inc. (see Page 270).

Seminars in Spain

Dr. Brenda Heinke of Seymour, Wisconsin, had decided to visit Spain in April 1986. She first planned to stay for five months, so that she could offer a course of five lectures. The first was to experienced behavioral optometrists who wished to expand their repertoire of practical visual training techniques. The rest were an extensive four-part series covering all aspects of functional optometry. The first was on the history of behavioral optometry and general binocular dysfunctions. The second was titled "Strabismus and Amblyopia." The third series covered developmental and perceptual vision and included the newer offshoots of optometric vision therapy such as sports vision, infant vision and the treatment of motion sickness. The fourth was completely practical: how to begin a practice that is devoted to optometric vision therapy and how to test and train the vision system.

All of the seminars that Dr. Heinke gave were in Madrid, and each of the two-day series lasted for a total of some fourteen hours. Many of the Spanish optometrists are members of the European Society of Optometry and the American Optometric Extension Program Foundation. Their response to Dr. Heinke's lectures was so strong that she prolonged her visit and started teaching classes to those optometrists in general practice who were interested in broadening the scope of their work to include optometric vision therapy.

A Clinic in Japan

After he had graduated from Dartmouth College in 1978, magna cum laude, Glen Swartwout followed in his father's footsteps and enrolled in a college of optometry. He graduated from the State University of New York's State College of Optometry in 1982 as Dr. Glen Swartwout, with a fistful of honors and the desire to make a substantial contribution to behavioral optometry before going into practice. Dr. Swartwout then spent the next two years as the first director of the Optometric Center of Tokyo, which he helped to found.

"Since World War II, the Westernization of Japan's education, as well as cultural, environmental and dietary changes have led to the growing presence of western-style problems in behavior and learning. Just as Japan is many decades behind America in the development of an optometric profession, it is certainly one or more decades ahead of us in its need for behavioral optometric care," Dr. Swartwout said, as he explained what had prompted him to spend 1983 and 1984 in Japan.

"Daily VDT users make up more than 25 percent of the work force in Tokyo. Participation in recreational sports is similarly high, with a tremendous emphasis upon performance. By the time a Japanese child reaches the age of three, she or he begins competitive formal schooling. From then through high school, children are under maximum academic load and stress, learning thousands of different symbols while competing for places in better schools. Even preschool entry is determined by intense preparation and oral exams.

"Japan has one of the highest literacy rates in the world, and industry and technology are highly advanced. Yet optometry as a profession lags behind that in the United States in many areas, legally, educationally, and clinically."

Dr. Swartwout helped to establish the Optometric Center of

Tokyo, an in-house research clinic for a major optical company, the Sanki Optical Group. Their support and that of the Kojima family of Tokyo made the project a reality.

"It will be several years before the clinic opens to the general public," Dr. Swartwout explained. "Marketing in Japan is very different from that in the States. It is extremely conservative and the companies want to be sure they will be successful with new ventures."

Under its new director, William Somers, Ph.D., O.D., who was on leave of absence from his duties as Chief of Indiana University's Vision Training Clinic, the center's objectives were to become financially self-sustaining while expanding its educational and research functions.

At the time of this book's publication, Japan has no legal recognition of optometry. Anyone can open an office or store and prescribe lenses; typically, the norm is for a refracting optician to have two years of training after graduating from high school; 90 percent of the refraction is done by unlicensed individuals. The one college is the Kikuchi College of Optometry in Nagoya. A dramatic difference from American standards, which demand a minimum of seven years of college education.

Since technically there are no Japanese optometrists, the description in Japan is "refracting optician." Most refracting opticians work for one of the large optical companies, with an ophthalmologist on site who evaluates eye health. The opticians fit and dispense lenses. Competition between optical companies is high and it is a tradition in Japan to try to be the best. Each store or office is usually in a commercial setting, such as a department store or large business center.

Japan's population is roughly half that of the United States, yet it supports the second largest cadre of "refracting opticians" in the world after the United States. Dr. Swartwout explains how a national characteristic subtly aids and abets the system.

"It is not acceptable to the national psyche to complain. The Japanese habit is to go to another store for another exam and another purchase of lenses or contacts if you are not comfortable with the first pair."

Dr. Swartwout spent two years in Japan. During that time, he spent many months of negotiation with the Japanese Ministry of Health seeking permission for optometric equipment to make its long journey by sea from the United States to Japan. Two bilingual optometric assistants were trained to smooth language and cultural differences. They also translated hundreds of pages of patient instructions for optometric vision therapy.

"The Japanese penchant for performance and positive intervention makes it possible for behavioral optometry to be a prize import. The Optometric Center of Tokyo is making good progress in filling its goal in bringing to Japan a valuable and much needed health therapy."

Sports Vision Travels Abroad

Perhaps not unexpectedly, this aspect of behavioral optometry may well be the practice with speedy growth. Amateur athletics are highly important in Japan. When the Japanese do embrace a new practice, they do it seriously. The Japanese culture is so homogeneous, that a product, idea or activity that catches on goes "big time." The Optometric Center of Tokyo has developed several systematic methods of visual training for sports vision, which have been favorably received.

In 1986, Tokyo Optical Company, Limited, the third largest optical company in Japan, invited Dr. Philip Smith of San Diego, a behavioral optometrist who practices sports vision, to come to Japan and share his experiences with athletes in the evaluation and training of their visual skills.

Dr. Smith worked with the manager and coach of the Hiroshima Carps Baseball team, winners of their division, similar to the American or National League Pennant. The

Carps were just starting on the World Series when their manager, Mr. Anan, met with Dr. Smith. Their minor league team trains with the Kansas City Royals team in Florida during spring training, and Mr. Anan was interested in developing a visual training program for them to use in the off season.

Dr. Smith worked with a number of Japanese refracting opticians, showing them how to test and train athletes' visual skills. The majority of vision testing and training will be done with the youth and young adults in the Hiroshima area.

Letters of praise

Health practitioners, regardless of the type of health care they practice, receive letters from grateful patients. Behavioral optometrists are no different. Dr. Lynn Hellerstein of Denver, Colorado, received the following letter in June 1978.

Dear Dr. Hellerstein:

I know that you would want to know the results of Peter's reading tests in May, administered by the Special Education Department of the Denver Public Schools. We are pleased and I know that you will be too.

Since you may want to keep this letter for your records, I will explain that Mrs. -----, special education teacher, worked with Peter one hour per school day during the school terms 1976-77 and 1977-78 on reading. In first grade, 1976-77, he made unsatisfactory progress and was only up to second grade performance in one of four areas of the Woodcock Reading Mastery Test. He began visual training in September of 1977 and therefore, on Wednesdays, was not in the special education class. I worked with him on the prescribed exercises 5-6 days per week out of 7.

He attended the vision therapy sessions for 45 minutes on Wednesday mornings September through March 1978.

The 1977-78 school term was spent in special education with much emphasis placed upon the word attack skills of reading as evidenced by Peter's 6.1 score in that section of the Woodcock Mastery.

I credit Peter's reading success this school term to the vision therapy program. Because of this program, Peter was able to be receptive to the re-enforcement of reading skills offered to him by the special education department. Peter is now phased out of special education and back to the regular classroom for the school term of 1978-79. A similar letter to this will be sent to the Denver Public Schools, appropriate department.

Dr. Hellerstein also received the following letter from an adult, who had benefited from therapy. Her case had been a difficult one and had presented severe problems, so much so that many optometrists might have been reluctant to embark on therapy that had such a low potential for success.

Dear Dr. Hellerstein:

I want you to know how much I appreciate all the help you have given me in the past 5 months. In fact, everyone in your office has been really nice to me and pleasant to deal with.

I really have never felt better in my life. The fact that I'm seeing better seems almost secondary by comparison. I feel like a tremendous weight has been lifted from my shoulders. It's amazing that "how" a person sees can open up a whole new world.

Being a teacher, I can really see how important the work you do is. I have experienced firsthand that vision is not only important to the general learning process but to the development of "self." I know that my experience here will help me keep an open eye and mind to kids that may be experiencing similar problems.

If you ever need someone to back up the importance or the effectiveness of what you are doing, please let me know. I'd be more than happy to share my views.

Thanks again for all your work and for taking a chance with me! I cannot express enough my gratitude.

In 1985, Dr. Robert Sanet of Lemon Grove, California, received the following letters:

Dear Dr. Sanet:

Thank you! Thank you! Thank you! It is exciting for us to come to the end of _____'s eye therapy, especially with the great progress he has made. When we started, _____ was having trouble with reading, spelling, eye-hand coordination, left and right distinction, ineffectiveness in sports and other challenges. He would work very hard in school and try his best in sports but would be very frustrated with the results he was getting. He didn't have much confidence in himself and would come home from school crying because he couldn't read and thought he was dumb.

Eye therapy gave us hope that what was causing his problems could be corrected. _____ worked hard at his home eye therapy assignments although many times it was a struggle and a frustration to him. Dr. Sanet and his excellent staff were very encouraging and gave us a lot of support. As time went along and things started to improve, so did _____'s attitude about himself and the importance of the eye therapy. It was a long hard struggle but the rewards were well worth it.

Because of eye therapy, _____ has made great gains. His reading, writing, and spelling have all improved to A's. He now has a batting average of over 500 in Little League and is playing forward in soccer and has made several goals this past season. Needless to say, his self-confidence and self-esteem have gone up tremendously. He is a very happy and cheerful little boy. His teacher said he set a great example in his class of not giving up but working on your challenges. Last Friday during closing ceremonies at school, _____ received an award

for being on the honor roll for both semesters. Eye
therapy has been a tremendous blessing in our lives.
Thank you, Dr. Sanet, and your super staff.

Dear Dr. Sanet:

I am writing you this letter in appreciation for what your
program has done for me and my son.
In the beginning I had reservations because I had never
heard anything about eye therapy but our optometrist
highly recommended you so I did what he asked and got
wonderful results.
I really couldn't see how you could cure my car sickness, headaches, or even my trouble with my balance,
not to mention my eyesight and eye control. You made a
believer out of me.
My son and I had the same basic problems but he was a
great deal worse. I have seen a great change in his school
work, sports and his attitude. My son and I both support
your program. It is great going through the mountains and
their winding roads and not getting car sick, and to work
all day without a headache.
We both enjoyed the sessions and the people we worked
with. We had a lot of fun doing the exercises. My husband is coming in next. He is really looking forward to
it, after seeing our results. Thanks!

Dear Dr. Sanet:

I'd like to thank all of you for the part you played in the
miracle of making my daughter a complete person.
We are so very thankful. _____ is so very happy, too.
You have taken a withdrawn child and a learning disabled child and made her see and feel like the rest of us.
I had tried hard to find help for her. I was worn out and
really didn't realize that you could solve so many of the
problems. Who would have believed that this could all

be helped in a few months - when I felt it might take a lifetime to help her.

She can now remember things she told you from minute to minute and day to day. I no longer feel she'll get lost a block from home.

You've truly given my daughter a whole new life to live. I can't thank each of you enough for being there and caring and helping her to become a happy, bubbly 10-year old. We were so desperate this time last year and so tired from trying to find some help for her.

Unique Philanthropy

The women and men who practice optometric vision therapy are uniquely qualified to help others. This they do, of course, in their practice of the therapy but many behavioral optometrist are also involved in community service. The scope of their activities is astonishingly varied and unpredictable. Here is a small random selection from the large number of philanthropic endeavors.

Dr. Tirsa Quinones, who grew up in Puerto Rico, has a full-time practice in New Haven, Connecticut, in which she specializes in vision therapy for youngsters and adults. She has helped develop a bilingual program for Spanish-speaking youngsters and originated a bilingual learning center for Spanish-speaking adults. Dr. Quinones has volunteered on a monthly basis at the Fair Haven Community Clinic to perform visual screenings--for the past twenty years. She also helped train and organize the founder members of the Connecticut Society for the Preservation of Vision.

Dr. Arnold Bierman of Lansdale, Pennsylvania, is another practitioner who has worked for years with community organizations. Dr. Bierman originated a visual screening program for the Jaycees, for which he taught volunteers how to register the children, take case histories and test for clarity of sight; once trained, the volunteers then assisted school nurses. In another aspect of this screening process, Dr. Bierman coordinated the work of interns from the Pennsylvania College of Optometry to handle additional vision screening. About 300 children were screened as a result of the project the first year, and the program has run periodically since then. As Dr. Bierman commented, "Although I saw very few new patients as a result of this project, I had been able to bring the concepts of behavioral optometry to a large group. I could never have run the project as an individual practitioner; the liaison with the Jaycees was beneficial to all."

Dr. Bierman was invited by the Director of Vision Services of the Montgomery Country Intermediate Unit to become the visual consultant for the preschool screening program. The director's daughter had been having great visual difficulties but had been told by ophthalmologists that "nothing was wrong" and it was "all in her head." When treated by Dr. Bierman with bifocals, the youngster's headaches stopped, her blurred vision cleared and her schoolwork improved. A few years later, Dr. Bierman was appointed visual consultant for the Pathway School, a school for students with learning disabilities and/or social or emotional adjustment problems. He has developed a comprehensive vision screening, which is now used routinely and provides lenses and training procedures when necessary.

Dr. Amorita Treganza is also well known for philanthropy and community activities in her California community of Lemon Grove. A practitioner of optometric vision therapy for over forty years, she has devoted more than three decades to working exclusively with children. In 1960 she was honored as San Diego's "Woman of Valor" ; in 1963, as San Diego's "Woman of the Year"; and in 1971, as San Diego's "Optometrist of the Year." In 1975, she received the Getman Award from the College of Optometrists in Vision Development, the highest honor possible in behavioral optometry. These honors were not only in recognition of her lectures and papers which are part of national study courses but also for the innumerable charitable contributions Dr. Treganza has made to her community. For eleven years she was with the Flying Samaritans, an organization which provided glasses for people in Baja. Then she volunteered with Project Amigos to provide glasses for people in Tijuana, Mexico. For many years, she has given free examinations and glasses to girls at a rehabilitation center near her practice.

Dr. Constantine Forkiotis, one of this book's coauthors, also is involved in community activities, only in his case, his community stretches across the United States. In 1971, Dr. Forkiotis was invited to address supervisory personnel at the Connecticut State Police. His talk, "Vision and Behavior Related to the Motor Vehicle Operator," piqued the interest of the Commissioner of the Connecticut State Police, who invited Dr. Forkiotis to use his expertise in working with the training officers at the academy.

The program with the State Police Department led to a request from the Police Explorer Section of the Boy Scouts of America to screen and educate scouts. Dr. Forkiotis also gives a great deal of time to working with municipalities around the country, helping them to learn about the background of the Horizontal Gaze Nystagmus test (HGN), which is used to detect drivers under the influence of alcohol or drugs. This aspect of his volunteer work has taken him to many different states, including Iowa, where in 1985 he presented an expert witness course to police training officers, state prosecuting attorneys, county attorneys and behavioral optometrists. Dr. Forkiotis has also been a consultant for the US Department of Transportation Research Office, the National Health Traffic Safety Administration for drug-testing detection and the National Standardized Behavioral Sobriety tests.

Behavioral Optometry Vital In Court Cases

At first, Dr. Forkiotis' role was to assist in the training of police officers to detect the HGN, which is the most accurate field test available to police officers checking on drug or alcohol intoxication of drivers. In the pamphlet "Optometric Expertise: The Scientific Basis for Alcohol Gaze Nystagmus," published by the Optometric Extension Program Foundation in April 1987, Dr. Forkiotis noted that over three thousand police officers have been trained to administer the behavioral tests involving vision and the visual mechanism.

While the program was in process, the court cases brought out an important question: establishment of the scientific proof of tests of the vision system by behavioral optometry. The Frye Amendment, Frye vs. United States, App. 1923 D.C., states that a procedure and process can not be admissible in the courtroom unless recognized and accepted by the scientific community.

"The judicial system was having difficulty finding expert testimony to back up the scientific basis of HGN in the courtroom, as required by law, even though HGN has been researched by various individuals from many aspects for over fifty years. In the courtroom, research and theory are not always sufficient. To win the case and establish the scientific basis, behavioral optometry by virtue of its philosophy, education, training, experience and daily practice of visual function and performance is the expert in HGN. I offered myself and my colleagues in behavioral optometry to assist in courtroom challenges," Dr. Forkiotis explains.

"The eyes offer virtually the best route to determine intoxication. When an individual is under the influence of alcohol or drugs, the central nervous system is suppressed. This suppression leads to the loss of control of the eyes. The eyes take on a jerky, oscillating movement. This is known as HGN.

"The explanation of HGN requires a dissertation of the basic philosophy of behavioral optometry. Thus far, behavioral optometry has saved a considerable amount of money for many states and municipalities. The Driving While Intoxicated/Horizontal Gaze Nystagmus (DWI/HGN) project is an extremely important public service effort for optometry as well as for our citizens and their safety. Tests available before DWI/HGN were not as reliable and often did not stand up in court. It was also possible for some people to cheat on the tests such as Walk and Turn and Stand on One Leg. It's impossible for anyone to cheat on DWI/HGN."

Dr. Forkiotis received the Homer Hendrickson Award in 1987. This award is presented annually by the Optometric Extension Program Foundation to an optometrist who has worked directly with organized community groups to solve community problems by applying behavioral vision care concepts. Certainly, by his many years of volunteer work in connection with DWI/HGN, Dr. Forkiotis has helped to make the roads in the United States safe for all.

Professional Organizations

The American Academy of Optometry (AAO) was founded in 1922 to foster the continued advancement of the education and knowledge of practicing optometrists. The academy publishes a monthly journal, the *American Journal of Optometry,* and *Physiological Optics.* In addition, it publishes educational articles and textbooks. It holds annual educational forums, offers postgraduate courses and encourages research and scientific investigations in optometry and related fields. The academy has a strict code of ethics and rigid standards of membership.

The American Optometric Association (AOA) represents more than 24,000 doctors of optometry and students of optometry. AOA was founded in 1898, and is a federation of local associations representing zones, states and the District of Columbia. A majority of the practicing optometrists in the United States are members. AOA publishes the *Journal of the American Optometric Association, AOA News* and a helpful selection of informative booklets for consumers and writers.

You can obtain publications from AOA by outlining your needs and sending them to:

The American Optometric Association
Communications Division
243 North Lindbergh Blvd.,
St. Louis, MO 63141

The Optometric Extension Program Foundation (OEP) is international in scope. It was founded in 1928 and is the principal provider of postgraduate education to optometrists. OEP publishes the *Journal of Behavioral Optometry*. The first organization to develop a wide variety of continuing educational courses for optometrist, OEP publishes pamphlets for the general reader. Among their most popular publications are:

"Does Your Child Have a Learning-Related Vision Problem?"

"VDTs and Vision: A User's Guide to Relieving Eyestrain, Headaches & Visual Stress"

"It's Never Too Late to Treat a Lazy Eye"

"What Is Visual Training?"

"Do You Have a Vision Problem?"

"Vision & Aging: Behavioral Vision Care Enriches Life After Age 40"

Write or call OEP for information and pamphlets. OEP also has a directory of optometrists, but if you call practitioners, always ask what type of optometry is practiced, since there is such a difference between general and behavioral optometry. (This is also the address for OEP's VisionExtension, Inc.)

The Optometric Extension Program Foundation
2912 South Daimler Street
Santa Ana, CA 92705
(714) 250-8070

The College of Optometrists in Vision Development (COVD) is a certifying body for practitioners of comprehensive functional eye care. Now an international organization, COVD was created in 1970 by a merger of behavioral optometric groups from around the United States.

COVD works with other professional organizations such as AOA, OEP, and the American Optometric Student Association and many concerned with providing maximum care for the public. They cooperate with the National Association for Children with Learning Disabilities, government agencies and many nonoptometric groups interested in related problems.

COVD publishes the *Journal of Optometric Vision Development*. In addition, COVD has created educational pamphlets for optometrists, professionals in health care, parents and educators.

The College of Optometrists in Vision Development
353 H Street, Suite C,
Chula Vista, CA 92010

Volunteers for Vision, Inc. This Texas-based organization was created in 1965 under the Community Action Program and Project Head Start. Its purpose is to instruct volunteers on how to conduct screening programs for 3-6 year olds. These programs may be at preschool centers, parochial schools, public schools or federally sponsored day care centers, wherever there is concern for the visual welfare of children. Their booklet, "A Manual of Instructions: A Guide for the Vision Screening of Children, is useful for individuals or groups and the organization's secretary is glad to discuss how to develop a screening program.

Volunteers for Vision, Inc.
P.O. Box 2211
Austin, TX 78768

Rehabilitation Services and Optometry Dr. Marla Moon, whose optometric practice is in State College, Pennsylvania, is also a consultant for a private agency, JMS Vision Loss Rehabilitation Inc., of Exton, Pennsylvania (a suburb of Philadelphia) and Boston, Massachusetts. The agency provides vision rehabilitation services for blind and visually impaired people of all ages in a variety of settings. A leader in the field of vision loss rehabilitation, JMS also has expertise in serving individuals with special needs, including the elderly, the multidisabled, and the retarded, whose amount of vision was unknown.

In the past, the conventional vision screening methods were used with such patients, usually with inaccurate results. JMS has developed a functional vision exam which accurately evaluates the vision of people who may have difficulty describing what they see. The benefits of the work JMS does with this population are profound. Formerly, most of the patients were given high doses of drugs. This left them capable of little more than lying on their beds. Visits to the bathroom, personal chores, even meals were events that required considerable help from the staff, for whom such involvement was a physical and emotional drain. Another aspect of the staff's work, that of dealing with people on drugs, was a potentially difficult, sometimes dangerous situation. Individual reactions cannot be foreseen and the stress and tension exacted a heavy toll.

In many cases, JMS has been highly successful in increasing the mobility and independence of their clients. On the basis of the extensive data gained from the visual analysis and treatment, individualized programs are designed for each patient. After these programs are developed, JMS then trains the staff at the institutions to give follow-up services.

The net gains are many. Patients have usually become capable of caring for themselves, and so become more active. They begin to feel good about themselves and have some self-confidence. In many cases, the use of drugs to control behavior is no longer necessary. Ultimately, the staff is released from the physical caretaking chores and able to provide the specialized help for which they are trained.

In Chapter 6, the work of Dr. William Padula is discussed. Services such as the Visually Impaired Program for Michigan's Oakland Intermediate School District, started in 1979 by an OEP study group and continuing under the aegis of optometrists S. Garmezana and P. Raznik are available throughout the U.S.; OEP or any of the American colleges of optometry are good referral sources.

Connecticut Society for the Preservation of Vision This group (CSPV) was founded in March 1983 by parents who had children with visual dysfunction that had not been identified as the underlying cause of learning differences and problems in school. A nonprofit group staffed by volunteers, its activities were initially funded by several grants. Its aim is to bring the public information about behavioral optometry and vision therapy. Their bylaws establish these goals:

1. Identify the visually disadvantaged person

2. Disseminate information on the importance of vision and options for proper care

3. Encourage and support research in vision

4. Provide resources and support to persons involved with visual welfare

The society holds informational meetings and will send members to speak to groups wishing to learn about optometric vision care. But they go beyond those basics. CSPV offers valuable public services that include instructional workshops and seminars, public meetings, parent support and advocate service in schools, a library information center and screenings, which are basic vision analyses for individuals or groups. They also train volunteers to handle comprehensive vision screenings. A complete screening includes evaluation, interpretation, consultations and recommendations, with follow-up consultations with schools or other professionals as needed. Founder members Linda de Francesco, B.S. Sp. Ed., Shirley Brog Kondo, B.S., Margie L. Rosenberg, B.S., OTR/L, and Henry E. Rosenberg, Ph.D., were themselves trained by behavioral optometrists Drs. C. Forkiotis, W. Padula and T. Quinones of Connecticut.

As an example of how the vision screenings of CSPV are used, the society was invited to the remedial learning center at the

University of New Haven for several years in a row to give vision screenings for several hundred students at the center. Not surprisingly, a high number of the students examined by the society had vision imbalances. Regretfully, the follow-through in such a situation is haphazard. Although society members make recommendations, it is the individual's prerogative to accept them or not. Youngsters in remedial education do not find it easy to initiate or cope with the schedule of going for regular office appointments for optometric vision therapy or doing home procedures. Even something which seems simple, wearing the lenses, may be really difficult for youngsters who are vulnerable to peer pressure. The society's legacy to the university was to train four instructors in vision screening methods.

Among their many accomplishments, the society has written a training manual specifically for the nonprofessional. CSPV has also developed a screening course which is available upon request. The course is about ten hours long, with five sessions of some two hours. Practice sessions are needed. Review courses are also offered. The group created screening procedures for the Headstart program in New Haven. In fact, in the spring of 1985, they screened 150 Headstart preschoolers.

The Parent Advocate   CSPV offers support and assistance to parents of learning-different children. The process helps to lessen the gap between the doctor's office and the school. This usually results in a good resolution of the child's problems.

"So many people called to say that their children were having trouble. Although often the schools had given testing, help was needed to plan for and obtain the appropriate services to fit the needs of the children," the society explains. One of their founder members has specific training with Connecticut Public Law 94-142, the basis for determining the rights of parents.

The society's goals are to continue its efforts to bring information to consumers as well as to train more volunteers to become vision screeners. It offers vision screenings whenever possible, at businesses, educational institutions, health fairs, even private homes--wherever requests take them. Write for information if you are interested in helping to establish a similar organization in your community.

The Connecticut Society for the Preservation of Vision
P. O. Box 7355
New Haven, CT 06519

Parents Active for Vision Education (PAVE) was founded in 1988 in San Diego, California. The president, Marjie Thompson, the parent of a child whose life was changed by vision therapy, has worked as a therapist since 1979 in the Lemon Grove, California, practice of Drs. Sanet, Hillier and Treganza. She gathered together other parents whose children had also suffered the effects of undetected performance-related vision problems to form the organization.

PAVE's purpose is to "raise awareness among children, parents, educators and the medical community of the critical relationship between vision and achievement." PAVE wants all children tested for the 4 F's (focusing, fusion, fixation, and form perception) before being taught the 3 R's. The group promotes and coordinates comprehensive performance related school vision screenings. They arrange lectures on vision and learning, stress relieving vision hygiene and how to structure the home and classroom for maximum visual learning. PAVE sponsored the first comprehensive vision education program in a San Diego school.

PAVE's monthly educational meetings are well attended and they are successful in their efforts to share news of the benefits of optometric vision therapy with parents, educators, psychologists, pediatricians and other professionals. If you are interested in establishing a PAVE chapter in your community contact:

Parents Active for Vision Education
National Headquarters

7331 Hamlet Avenue
San Diego, CA 92120

Recommended Reading and Viewing

The general reader doesn't have a wide choice of books about behavioral optometry. From the vast array of professional books for practitioners, Dr. Arnold Gesell's book, *Vision -- Its Development in Infant and Child,* is the fruit of almost a decade of intense work by a team of experts. It paved the way for the probing research into the connection between behavior and vision by the Gesell Institute's Department of Vision, but although clearly written, it is aimed primarily at professionals in health care and education. First published in 1949, *Vision* does not have any information on the subsequent development and practice of behavioral optometry; nevertheless it is an illuminating introduction to the origins of this innovative health care.

In contrast, two books by Dr. Richard Kavner, *Total Vision* and *Your Child's Vision,* are aimed at the general reader. They contain a wealth of valuable information about behavioral optometry and also offer helpful material on health, nutrition, and children's development.

Either of these books can be ordered from OEP's Vision Extension, Inc.

Dr. Robert-Michael Kaplan is the author of a fascinating book, *Seeing Beyond 20/20,* which can be supplemented by audio tapes. Dr. Kaplan suggests ways and means to reduce stress on your vision system and to learn to use your vision well.

Seeing Beyond 20/20 was published in 1987 by Beyond Words Publishing, Route 3, Box 492B, Hillsboro, OR 97123, and costs $12.95. Write to Vision Alternatives, P. O. Box 25412, Portland, OR 97225, for information or to order the audio tapes "Relax and See," self-guided imagery ($11.95 + $2.50 for handling) and "21-day Vision Games," 3 audio tapes ($49.95 + $2.50 for handling).

In 1987, the Optometric Extension Program Foundation

(OEP) established a division, VisionExtension, Inc., to handle the sale of informational materials relating to behavioral optometry.

Their catalog, which is updated regularly, contains items of vision therapy equipment (usually for the use of the behavioral optometrist), video and audio tapes, and an interesting selection of books. The catalog material listed will probably be of value to many different professionals in related health fields such as social work, education and psychology. It also has videos, such as the one by the Kansas Optometric Association. This two-part video (each part lasts 17 minutes) covers the development of vision from infancy and shows the visual problems that arise from classroom tasks. It is ideally suited for viewing by parents, educators, and groups concerned with learning about vision and optometric vision therapy. If you want a copy of the catalog, write VisionExtension, Inc., 2912 South Daimler Street, Ste. 100, Santa Ana, CA 92705.

"The Mind's Eye; The Experience of Learning." This documentary, made by professionals, came out in 1986 under the aegis of the Walt Disney Company. Screenwriter Alvin Sargent, who has received two academy awards for his scripts, which include "Ordinary People," "Julia," and "Paper Moon," was a patient of behavioral optometrist Dr. Moses Albalas of Los Angeles for about six months, a time which brought radical differences to this gifted writer.

"The therapy changed the way I perceived my life," commented Mr. Sargent. "Up to then, I wasn't a fighter. I usually gave in. But I found myself seeing with both eyes after the therapy. Actually, the therapy is about identity. When you realize what the therapy is, you want to share the news with everyone. I brought the idea for a documentary to Disney and they found producer Terri Strauss." The documentary includes other therapies for the learning disabled and, in addition to some 15 minutes that featured Alvin Sargent in therapy at the Los Angeles office of Dr. Albalas, it shows Bruce Jenner, Oliver Reed and Harvey Korman with his son Chris who had dyslexia.

"The Mind's Eye" was first featured on the Disney channel in March of 1986 and has been shown subsequently.

Some of the books listed below are not easily available. If your bookstore does not carry them or cannot order them, try your library. Remember interlibrary loan may turn up a copy elsewhere if your local library does not have the title in its catalog card.

Bartley, S. Howard. *The Human Organism as a Person, The Principles of Optometry.* Radnor, PA: Chilton, 1967.
This book, by a professor of psychology at the Laboratory for the study of Vision and Related Sensory Processes, Michigan State University, bridges the gap between biology and psychology and is of value to optometrists, ophthalmologists, psychologists, biologists, anthropologists and educators. Professor Bartley, a National Research Council Fellow in the 1930s, also served as Professor of Research in Visual Sciences and as Director of Research for the Office of Scientific Research and Development at the Dartmouth Medical School Eye Institute.

Dawkins, H. Richmond, Edelman, E. and Forkiotis, C. *Suddenly Successful Student, A Guide to Overcoming Learning & Behavior Problems.* Available from VisionExtension, Inc.

Friedman, E. and Lulow, K. *Dr. Friedman's Vision Training Program.* New York: Bantam Books, 1983.

Gesell, Arnold, Ilg, Francis L. and Bullis, G. E. *Vision--Its Development in Infant and Child.* New York: Harper & Row, 1971 [1st ed., 1949]. Available from VisionExtension, Inc.

Getman, G. N. *How to Develop Your Child's Intelligence.* Irvine, CA: Research Publications, 1982 [orig. pub. 1958]. Available from VisionExtension, Inc.

Gilman, G. *Behavioral Optometry,* Quincy, CA: Paradox Publishing, Box 3590. Available from VisionExtension, Inc.

Gregory, R. L. *Eye and Brain.* New York: World University Library/McGraw-Hill, 1966.

Huxley, Aldous. *The Art of Seeing.* Berkeley, CA: Creative Arts Book Company. [1st edition by Harper & Row, 1942].

Hoopes, A. and T. *Eye Power.* New York: Knopf, 1979.

Kavner, R. and Dusky, L. *Total Vision.* New York: A. and W. Publishers, 1979. Available from VisionExtension, Inc.

Kavner, R. *Your Child's Vision, A Parent's Guide to Seeing, Growing, and Developing.* New York: Simon & Schuster Inc., 1985. Available from VisionExtension, Inc.

Padula, W. *Behavioral Optometric Approaches in Vision Care for Persons with Physical Disabilities.* Santa Ana, CA: Vision Extension, Inc., 1988.

Seidermann, A. and Schneider, S. *The Athletic Eye.* New York: Hearst, 1983.

Solan, H. A., ed. *The Treatment & Management of Children with Learning Disabilities.* Springfield, IL: Charles C. Thomas, 1982.

Streff, J., Ames, L. B. and Gillespie, J. *Stop School Failure.* New York: Harper & Row, 1972.

Helpful Periodicals

The professional journals such as *The Journal of Behavioral Optometry,* the *Journal of the American Optometric Association, American Journal of Optometry* and *Physiological Optics* and the *Journal of Learning Disabilities* all have excellent articles. Your optometrist may have copies which you can borrow, or have your library make an interlibrary loan, if possible, from one of the colleges of optometry.

Perhaps the clearest material for the consumer is that published by the American Optometry Association, particularly AOA's *Optometric Care Advice for Infants and Children News Backgrounder* and *Vision Therapy News Backgrounder,* and the many pamphlets, such as "Spelling: A Visual Skill" and those listed earlier from the Optometric Extension Program Foundation. You'll find addresses in the previous section dealing with these organizations. If you are buying in quantity, ask for group rates.

Glossary

Accommodation   An important visual skill which allows us to see clearly at all distances.

Amblyopia   This is also known as "lazy eye" and with this situation, sight is below the expected, normal level. Amblyopia results from a problem with the function of the vision system, such as early strabismus or nystagmus.   The brain quickly learns to suppress, or shut off the processing of input through the "lazy" eye's circuit.   Amblyopia *at any age* can usually be successfully treated by optometric vision therapy.   About 2 percent of the general population has it.

Astigmatism   The development of unequal curvature of the cornea.   Thus, the light gathered in by the eye is not focused properly.

Binocularity   The simultaneous use of the two eyes in the act of vision.

Binocular vision   The type of vision in which the two eyes are related in their movements so that they are both directed at the same point of regard and each contributes simultaneously to the total perception.

Compensating lens,   see Minus lens (concave) and Plus lens.

Convergence   The act of turning the two eyes inward, toward each other, in order to see a near object. You might be reading or watching a ball move.

Coordination   The two eyes working together in binocular vision; this is also known as teaming.

Cornea   The transparent portion on the front of the eyeball, over the iris and pupil.

Depth perception   Perception of the relief of objects in which they appear to be in three dimensions rather than as flat pictures (see Stereopsis).

Dominant eye   In optometric vision therapy, this is generally described as the "preferred eye." An individual is usually consistent in using the same eye for all responses; it is a response of the motor system, during which the individual aligns either eye toward the object of regard. The preferred eye response usually matches handedness.

Esophoria   A tendency for one or both eyes to run in (over-converge) beyond the expected while looking at objects at various distances. The eye(s) will look straight but special tests reveal the tendency to cross.

Esotropia   Also known as an internal squint, in which one or both eyes turn inward (crossed eyes) and can be observed cosmetically.

Exophoria   A tendency for one or both eyes to turn out. Keep in mind that this describes a tendency and therefore the eyes will look cosmetically straight. However, tests will reveal the tendency to turn out.

Exotropia   One or both eyes may turn out, away from one another; this is also known as external squint (wall eyed) and can be observed cosmetically.

Extraocular muscles   The six muscles that guide movement of the eye: internal and external recti, superior and inferior recti, and superior and inferior oblique. The brain *controls* the voluntary nervous system and thus *controls* eye movements; the muscles *direct* eye movements.

Farsightedness   See hyperopia.

Fixation   Aiming or directing the eyes while shifting rapidly from one object to another, such as reading from word to word on a line, or copying from a textbook to a notebook.

Focus This function of the vision system identifies information gathered through fixations. The ability of the focusing mechanism to change quickly and accurately while exerting the least amount of energy depends on the individual's stress response. The focusing response is under the control of the involuntary nervous system (autonomic); however, it is possible to gain some control over the focusing function through certain optometric vision therapy procedures that use biofeedback, or internal awareness of bodily functions.

Form sense, form perception The ability to organize and recognize visual sensations as shapes, noticing likes and differences (such as the difference between *was* and *saw, that* and *what*. This ability depends on eye movements used during fixations and eye scanning of the visual space around us.

Fusion A binocular response that simultaneously combines the separate inputs from the two eyes into a single mental image at the brain level (the visual cortex).

Hyperopia (farsightedness) A refractive condition of the eye in which an object can be seen clearly only by using extra accommodation. Small amounts are normal.

Iris The colored ring surrounding the eye's pupil.

Lens A transparent, flexible medium with two boundary surfaces, one of which is curved.

Macula The area at the center of the retina which has clearest vision. The macula contains only cones and does not have any rods.

Minus lens (concave) A lens used traditionally by both ophthalmologists and general optometrists (non-behavioral optometrists) to compensate for myopia. This type of lens compresses the space world, increases the strain on the muscles and encourages rigidity, and thus less flexibility, of both physical movement and mental problem-solving.

Myopia Commonly called *nearsightedness*. A symptom of a vision imbalance; the myopic individual has difficulty seeing distant objects clearly.

Nasal occluders (nasal or binasal tapes) In the 1950s, California optometrist Dr. Louis Jaques published a book, *Corrective and Preventive Optometry*. In it, he discussed procedures in which he used "half covers" for the treatment of strabismus. Since then, the use of nasal occluders has become widespread in optometric vision therapy. The width of the tape applied to the spectacles varies, depending on the effect desired. The tapes "disrupt" the wearer's customary visual habits. You are forced to change how you "load your retina with light." It is virtually impossible for you to continue to view the world in the way you adapted to out of need.

As well as treating strabismus, the tapes are useful with amblyopia and suppression. Nasal tapes are also used successfully to: persuade the individual who relies almost exclusively on their central vision to start using more peripheral information; treat a myopic individual whose style is to constrict space and ignore a great deal of peripheral information; attempt to change the direction of an individual's inwardization, or self-gratification, so that they become more empathetic and outgoing; to expand one's space world so that one develops the ability to handle both central and peripheral information simultaneously; and to increase one's reading ability so that you can take in larger amounts of information in a given period of time.

Nystagmoid oscillation An undulating, vibratory movement of one or both eyes; the oscillation is usually of equal speed and amplitude in each direction. One type of motion is pendular and may be seen in either the horizontal, vertical, diagonal or rotary direction; a second type is a jerky, rhythmic (or spring type) movement in one direction followed by a rapid return to the original position; this may be observed in horizontal, vertical, diagonal, rotary clockwise or counterclockwise direction. The second type of motion occurs as the result of alcohol or drug use; police officers are trained to test drivers for this type of motion if drivers are suspected of being intoxicated. **Note:** Police officers may only stop a motorist when they have due cause and reason. It is estimated that some four percent of the population have a nystagmoid oscillation occurring naturally, without the use of alcohol or drugs. Generally, these individuals will know of their handicap and will either have restricted licenses or be able to inform the police of the situation.

Optic nerve The main nerve to the eye; this nerve connects the eye to seeing part of the brain.

Plus lens A lens traditionally used by both ophthalmologists and general optometrists (non-behavioral optometrists) to compensate for hyperopia (farsightedness). It has the opposite effect of a minus lens (see glossary). In addition to the conventional use of the plus lens, the behavioral optometrist uses it to remediate or nurture an immature vision system and change behavioral responses. Plus lenses are also used as part of optometric vision therapy programs. These lenses are very effective in helping an individual keep their visual system in balance.

Pupil The opening in the center of the eye through which light passes into the eye.

Refraction The clinical measurement of the eye to determine the need for lenses; in behavioral optometry this is only one part of the visual analysis to determine the need for lenses.

Retina The innermost layer of the eye. This is a layer of complex nerve endings upon which light rays are focused; it contains the rod and cone cells.

Retinoscope A hand-held instrument used by professionals in eye care to measure, objectively, the refractive situation.

Sight The ability to focus and see both at distance and near. The clarity depends on the flexibility of the focusing system and is only one aspect of vision.

Snellen chart A chart on which lines of symbols (letters and numbers) are printed in graded sizes. The largest symbols are at the top of the chart. Devised over one hundred years ago, the only visual skill the eye chart tests is how clearly you see at a distance of twenty feet.

Stereopsis The visual perception of three dimensions or depth. Generally, the term is applied to depth perception that results from having two eyes separated horizontally so that each eye sends in visual information from a different angle. We use stereopsis to determine the relative distances between objects by looking at them from two difference places (the two eyes) simultaneously.

Strabismus A condition where one eye fixes on an object and the other eye points in another direction. About five percent of the general population has strabismus, which is also described as heterotropia, crossed eyes, squint and walleye.

Suppression The process in which all or part of the visual input of one eye is prevented from contributing to the binocular perception. When we use both eyes to see, and combine the information received through each eye to make one mental picture at the brain level, we have binocular vision; if we use just one eye and mentally shut off the input from the other eye, we do not have binocular vision--it is suppressed. Failure to develop the equal, "teamed" use of both eyes together, in a binocular way, can lead to such symptoms as word reversals; it also can restrict development in terms of gross and fine motor skills and reduces one's ability to solve problems.

Teaming ability The skill of accurately aiming both eyes together as a paired team while scanning in all directions. In technical terms, this is binocularity. Some youngsters and adults can team their eyes fairly well when looking in the distance but have a difficult time teaming when trying to read or work at near, such as reading or computers. Their eyes fail to stay teamed momentarily, which causes double vision or may lead to suppression (this is then described as an avoidance reaction).

Vision, central This gives us optimum clarity when we read, play sports, look at objects. Central vision is limited in that we only see small amounts of information in a given period.

Vision, field of The area over which vision is possible, including motion, relative position of objects in space, contrast and movement sensitivity in side vision (reading from line to line without getting lost on the page).

Vision, peripheral We also call this side vision. Peripheral vision includes left, right, far, near, above and below. Peripheral vision enables us to keep our place as we read or walk. Infants use this visual skill early in life to judge distance and learn about size. Poorly developed peripheral vision can lead to symptoms such as being "accident prone," losing one's place when reading, poor copying ability, bumping into objects--generally lowering our ability to move efficiently.

Visual discrimination The ability to detect small differences in forms.

Visual memory The ability to recall within four or five seconds all the characteristics of a given form and being able to find this form from a selection of similar forms (short-term memory or immediate recall).

Visual perception The capacity to give meaning to what is seen. It is recognition, insight and interpretation at the cortical, or brain, level of what is seen.

Appendix I

TYPICAL PROFESSIONAL PROGRAMS IN OPTOMETRY[1], DENTISTRY[2], AND MEDICINE[3]

First Two Years

OPTOMETRY	DENTISTRY	MEDICINE
Histology	Histology	Histology
Physiology	Physiology	Physiology
Gross Anatomy	Gross Anatomy	Gross Anatomy
Cell Biology		Cell Biology
	Biochemistry	Biochemistry
Microbiology	Microbiology	Microbiology
General Pharmacology	Pharmacology	Pharmacology
General Pathology	Pathology	General & Systemic Pathology
Neurosciences	Neuroanatomy	Neuroscience
Neurophysiology		
		Neurochemistry
		Neuropathology
		Intro to Clinical Neurology
Nutrition	Nutrition	
Public Health	Behavioral Sciences and Community Health	Behavioral Sciences
Human Development		
	Inheritance & Devlpmt.	Genetics
	Principles of Human Behavior	
		Human Sexuality
	Humanities	
		Epidemiology
		Medical Ethics
Clinical Diagnosis	Physical Diagnosis	Physical Diagnosis
Ocular Anatomy		
	Materials Science	
Human Vision		
		Embryology
Ocular Physiology		
	Normal Mastication	
Ocular Biochemistry		
		Immunology
Ocular Pathology		
	Life support & Cardio Pulmonary Resuscitation	
		Intro to Clinical Sciences
Perceptual Devlpmt.		
		Parasitic Diseases
Geometric Optics		
Physiological Optics		
Visual Perception		
Physical Opticss		
Binocular Vision		
Refractive Error		
Strabismus & Amblyopia		
Accommodation, Convergence		
Contact Lenses		
Ophthalmic Optics		
Optometric Methods (includes beginning patient care)		

Third Year

OPTOMETRY	DENTISTRY	MEDICINE

OPTOMETRY

Ocular Pharmacology

Contact Lenses

Functional Visual Analysis

Vision Training

Geriatric Optometry

Behavioral Vision Analysis

Care of the Partially Sighted

Ocular Pathology
Ophthalmic Optics

Epidemiology

Behavior modification

Tests and Measurements

Public Health

Clinical Methods
  (11 hours pe week
  of supervised
  patient care at
  the University
  Optometric Center

DENTISTRY

General and Oral Medicine

Detection & Treatment of Oral and Facial Cancer

Cardiology

Behavioral Sciences

Community Health

Clinical Pathology

Humanities

Endodontics
Fixed Prosthodontics

Occlusion

Operative Dentistry

Oral and Maxillifacial surgery

Oral Diagnosis

Orthodontics

Pedodontics

Pedodontics

Radiology
Removable Prostho-
  dontics
Nutrition

MEDICINE

CLINICAL CLERKSHIPS
(Bedside Instruction)

Surgical

Obstetrical and Gynecological

Medical

Pediatric

Psychiatric and Neurological

Fourth Year

Bioelectronics
(elective)

Senior Research
(elective)

Contact Lenses

Illumination
(elective)

Emergency Care

Psychodynamics of patient care

Behavior Modifica-
tion Practicum

Special Testing
(elective)

Family Practice Program

Elective courses in Basic and Clinical Services

Two-month Junior Internship in specific Clinical
Disciplines at NYU School of Medicine

Remaining 6 months:

Free Elective Period
Research or clinical
Programs at scienti-
fic institutions and
hospitals in US and
abroad

Practice Administra-
tion
Clinical Care Study
Seminar

Research Methods

Ocular Pathology

Developmental
Disabilities

Public Health

Learning Disabilities

Clinical Internships
- (20 hours per week of supervised clinical care
on patients at the University Optometric Center)

1. State University of New York, State College of Optometry Catalog 1984-86. Pg. 64.

2. New York University Bulletin 12984-85, College of Dentistry. Pg. 18.

3. New York University School of Medicine, 1986, Information for Applicants. Pg. 3.

Appendix II

GUEST EDITORIAL
DISCREDITING THE BASIS OF THE AAO POLICY
LEARNING DISABILITIES, DYSLEXIA, AND VISION
Nathan Flax, O.D.
Rochelle Mozlin, O.D.
Harold A. Solan, O.D.

In 1972, the American Academy of Pediatrics, the American Academy of Ophthalmology and Otolaryngology, and the American Association of Ophthalmology issued a policy statement entitled "The Eye and Learning Disabilities," which denied any relationship between vision and learning. Flax[1] pointed out the gross distortions and inaccuracies in the use of reference materials which accompanied the position paper, concluding that "the dissemination of this statement . . . does a disservice to the public and represents an affront to the academic community."

An ad hoc working group of the American Association for Pediatric Ophthalmology and Strabismus and the American Academy of Ophthalmology recently issued a policy statement entitled "Learning disabilities, Dyslexia, and Vision,"[2] offering conclusions similar to those in the 1972 paper. Since these prestigious and scholarly organizations have put forth such dogmatic statements regarding the role of vision in learning disabilities, the authors thought a careful examination of the position paper and its fifteen references was warranted.

Analysis of supporting citations

A synopsis of the position paper is included in Appendix III, page 289. The following is an analysis of its supporting citations. We find that the gross distortions and inaccuracies in the 1972 statement still prevail.

The position paper uses three citations to support the statement that "children with learning disabilities have the same incidence of ocular abnormalities (e.g., refractive errors and muscle imbalance, including nearpoint convergence and binocular fusion abilities) as children without." These references warrant a closer look.

Flax's paper[1] never mentions incidence, but it does point out that refractive error and visual acuity do not correlate with learning ability or scholastic success. The thrust of the article is to differentiate the types of visual factors that do relate to learning and reading. Deficiencies in several visual functions (binocular fusion, accommodation, ocular motilities) contribute to reading inefficiency, poor comprehension, and discomfort. However, these factors cannot be responsible for a total inability to learn to read. In some instances, a visual perceptual disability makes it difficult to develop word recognition skills.

Bettman, Stern, Whitsell, and Gofman[2] are also used to support the statement that no differences exist in incidence of visual problems in children with learning disability as compared to normals. They compared 47 dyslexic children (diagnosed by the Pediatric Child Study Unit of the University of California San Francisco Medical Center) to 58 good readers of the same age and grade. Measurements of refractive error and nearpoint of convergence are not reported, yet this paper is cited to support the statement that no differences exist between the two groups in these areas. Some important differences were revealed in other aspects of visual function. They state:

> Yet, 42% of the dyslexic children had foveal suppression detected by the four-diopter prism test at distance or near, compared with 9% of the controls. This difference is highly significant statistically ($x^2 > 14$) and may indicate another neuromuscular abnormality frequently present in dyslexia.

> Fifty-two percent of dyslexic children showed gross jerkiness of their eyes in attempting to follow a pencil

tip moved along a diagonal line. Only 11% of the
controls had such jerkiness. The difference between
the two groups was readily apparent to the observer
and is highly significant statistically ($x^2 = 6.9$). This
may be another manifestation of defective fine motor
coordination.

Apparently, the committee which prepared this policy statement did not read their own references very carefully. If they
had, the Bettman et al, article would have been excluded, since
it seems to point out significant differences in visual function
between normally achieving and dyslexic children.

The article by Norn, Rindziunski, and Skydsgaard [3] goes to
great lengths to differentiate between primary reading retarda-
tion, or specific dyslexia, and secondary reading problems,
which can be attributed to intelligence defects, brain damage,
or exogenous factors. The term "specific dyslexia" is reserved
for those cases where all these secondary factors have been
ruled out, leaving a hereditary organic brain defect which can
be referred to a dysfunction in the patient's parietal-occipital
zone. So rigid is their interpretation of the term "specific
dyslexia" that they state "if cure is obtained, this must be due
to a mistaken diagnosis." By definition, visual anomalies are
excluded as a cause of specific dyslexia, but are acknowledged
as potentially making the situation worse.

The data support the conclusion that the incidence of refractive error is equal among the two populations, but other statements are worthy of citation. The dyslexic children had a
greater incidence of both subjective complaints associated with
near work and latent strabismus (defined as an exophoria
greater than 6 years below grade level to a neuropsychiatric
disorder related to metabolic abnormalities of the biogenic
amines. Most research into the etiology of dyslexia and application of research findings to clinical management is
hampered by lack of a consistent operational definition of
dyslexia or learning disability. Keogh [4] astutely points out that
"the controversy surrounding a developmental vision therapy

program probably reflects the current state of the art in learning disabilities." Rather than identifying this as a potential point of confusion, the policy statement avoids defining terms. Whether this ambiguity is intentional or demonstrates lack of understanding of the issue is unclear.

This policy statement of the American Academy of Ophthalmology and the American Association for Pediatric Ophthalmology and Strabismus does the public a disservice. It draws sweeping generalizations aimed at optometry with no conclusive supporting documents. The references offered are misconstrued, nonapplicable and grossly distorted. The same references can be used to support vision therapy as a treatment mode for learning-disabled children (in properly selected cases). The dissemination of this policy statement is an affront to the academic community and can only be viewed as such by the many disciplines which honestly serve the learning-disabled child.

Evaluation of the learning-disabled child is traditionally multidisciplinary. It is important to deal with any defect or problem that may be either causal or contributory to the child's problem. The policy statement itself supports the intervention necessary to correct any such problem. It is therefore illogical for the ad hoc committee not to endorse vision therapy as a necessity in those cases where defects in visual function such as binocular fusion, accommodation, and ocular motor deficiencies interfere with the ability to respond to educational remediation.

State University of New York
State College of Optometry
100 East 24th Street
New York, NY 10010

REFERENCES
1. Flax N. Visual function in learning disabilities, J Learning Disabilities, 1:551, Sept. 1968.

2. Bettmen JW Jr, Stern EL, Whitsell LJ, Gofman HF. Cerebral dominance in developmental dyslexia: Role of Ophthalmology, Arch. of Ophthalmology, 78:722-730, Dec. 1967.

3. Norn MS. Rindziunsky, and Skydsgaard, Ophthalmologic and orthoptic examinations of dyslectics, Acta Ophthalmologica, 47:147, 1969.

4. Keogh B. Optometric vision training programs for learning disability children: Review of issues and research, presented, in part, at the 10th annual meeting of the Association for Children with Learning Disabilities, March 15, 1973, Detroit, Michigan.

Appendix III

SYNOPSIS OF THE 1981 AMERICAN ACADEMY OF OPHTHALMOLOGY POLICY STATEMENT ON LEARNING DISABILITIES, DYSLEXIA AND VISION

The statement paper published in 1981 (and by 1991 no change in the Academy's position had emerged) explains that the policy of the American Academy of Ophthalmology and the American Association for Pediatric Ophthalmology and Strabismus is to support the position that a child or adult with dyslexia or a related learning disability should receive:

a. early medical, educational, or psychological evaluation and diagnosis.

b. treatment with educational procedures or proven value, demonstrated by scientifically valid research.

After commenting on the background of dyslexia and related learning disabilities, the statement notes that: "Dyslexia and related learning disabilities, as well as other forms of learning under-achievement, require a multidisciplinary approach from medicine, education, and psychology in evaluation, diagnosis, and treatment."

Then the Academy states that, "Eye care should never be instituted in isolation when a person does have dyslexia or a related learning disability. Children identified as having such problems should be evaluated for general medical, neurologic, psychologic, visual, and hearing defects. If any problems of this nature are found, they should be corrected as early as possible."

They make the point that since clues in word recognition are transmitted through the eyes to the brain, it has, "unfortunately, become common practice to attribute reading difficulties to subtle ocular abnormalities, presumed to cause faulty perception. Although eyes are necessary for vision, the brain encodes information resulting in visual perception."

Then comes what is probably the most important sentence in the entire statement: "Attention directed to the eyes would not be expected to have any effect on the brain's processing of visual stimuli." If this is the case, why would we bother to wear glasses at all? If you do not see clearly, how can you understand what you see, whether it is reading, shopping or playing sports? We know that putting glasses on helps our brain interpret the information. If one method, putting on glasses, is acceptable, how does it suddenly become the only valid method? Why discount other methods such as optometric vision therapy, given that it usually includes lens use? Above all, one asks if it is wise or appropriate to "disconnect" the eyes from the brain, as the academy suggests we do.

Throughout the statement, optometric research is cited but the reader is asked to believe that the research is not valid. The summation of the statement is that any vision therapy is mis-leading, since it may create a false sense of security. The work of behavioral optometry is literally dismissed. Believe what you are told to believe. Is this reminiscent of the *Emperor's New Clothes*?

Appendix IV

THE NIM TECHNIQUE

One of many ways to help individuals learn to read, the "Neurological Impress Remedial Reading Technique," (NIM) by R. S. Hockelman, Ph.D., is available in reprint No. 103 from *Academic Quarterly,* Vol. 1, No. 4. Specialists in remedial education will have other suggestions for ways to help.

NIM is an economical and time-saving method for working on remedial reading (only outlined here, discuss with tutor or obtain reprint). Its simplicity often makes people doubt its value and efficiency. Careful trial and experimentation has shown that NIM is effective and often superior to other methods. It is low cost and simple to use. If the individual does not respond to NIM after approximately four hours of use, then it's more than likely that it is not the method of choice for this particular person and another technique might be more appropriate.

Several studies were made of NIM, the first in 1961, another in 1963, a third in 1965. The students ranged from grade 6-10 and all showed significant increases in reading levels, often in short times. The student discussed in this book, Dr. Friedel's patient in Tucson, was a 5th grader and the technique was used for 15 minutes a day, on consecutive days, for about 8 hours. Improvement came at the end of the 8 hours; it was necessary to repeat the technique about six months later, in the next grade, when the youngster again seemed to be struggling with reading.

The technique is a multisensory approach and is most effective when used one on one, although a group setting is workable -- with earphone use for the students and a microphone for the tutor. It is preferable for the instructor to sit slightly behind the individual being tutored, so that the tutor's voice is close to the student's ear. From the first session, the instructor and student read the same material out loud together. Despite any mistakes, the student is advised to try to keep up with the instructor.

As the author of this method notes, many people do not read well because of a malfunctioning of the eye movements. Thus, the NIM method uses certain tactics to help the reader integrate smooth eye movement with the verbal work of reading aloud. The tutor does not at any time ask the student what is being read or test for word recognition or reading comprehension. The major concern is with the style rather than accuracy of reading.

This method is a type of audio-neural conditioning which works to replace the incorrect reading habits with correct, fluid habits. The reprint also notes that a copious supply of reading material is needed. It suggests that if after four hours, the individual is not responding, consider changing to kinesthetic or motor methods or to another technique called "echoing." The latter might be used as a supplemental technique with NIM and more intensively with those with auditory discrimination problems.

Appendix V

SCIENTIFIC STUDIES

This small selection is from a wealth of reputable scientific studies which establish the efficiency of behavioral optometric vision care. A full bibliography is in "The Efficacy of Visual Therapy: Accommodative disorders and Non-Strabismic Anomolies of Binocular Vision," Part I of III, by Drs. I. Suchoff and G. T. Petito, in the *Journal of the American Optometric Association,* 1986. Scientific studies are reviewed in the professional journals in "Helpful Periodicals." The *Journal of the College of Vision Development* also publishes bibliographies of studies.

Bachara, G. H., and Zaba, J. N. "Learning disabilities and juvenile delinquency: Beyond the correlation." *J. Learning Disabilities* 2(4), April 1978.

Birnbaum, M., Koslowe, K., Sanet, R. "Success in amblyopia therapy as a function of age: A literature review." *Am. J. Optom. & Physiol. Opt.* 54(4):269-275, 1977.

Ciuffreda, K. J., Kenyon, R. V., Stark, L. "Different rates of functional recovery of eye movements during orthoptic treatment in an adult amblyope." *Invest. Opthal. & Vis. Sci.* 18(2):213-219, 1979.

Ciuffreda, K. J., Goldrich, S. G., Neary, C. "Use of eye movement auditory biofeedback in the control of nystagmus." *Am. J. Optom. & Physiol. Opt.* 59(5):396-409, 1982.

Cooper, J., Selenow, A., Ciuffreda, K. J., Feldman, J., Faverty, J., Hokoda, S., Silver, J. "Reduction of aesthenopia in patients with convergence insufficiency after fusional vergence training." *Am. J. Optom. & Physiol. Opt.* 60(12):982-989, 1983.

Daum, K. "The course and effect of visual training on the vergence system." *Am. J. Optom. & Physiol. Opt.* 59(3):223-227, 1982.

Daum, K. "Accommodative insufficiency." *Am. J. Optom. & Physiol. Opt.* 60(5):352-359, 1983.

Flax, N., Duckman, R. "Orthoptic treatment of strabismus." *J. Amer. Optom. Assoc.* 49(12):1353-1360, 1978.

Goldrich, S. "Optometric therapy of divergence excess strabismus." *Am. J. Optom. & Physiol. Optics* 57(1):7-14, 1980.

Goldrich, S. "Oculomotor biofeedback therapy for exotropia." *Am. J. Optom. & Physiol. Optics* 59(4):306-317, 1982.

Hoffman, L., Cohen, A., Feur, G., Klayman, L. "Effectiveness of optometric therapy for strabismus in a private practice." *Am. J. Optom. & Physiol. Opt.* 47(12):990-995, 1970.

Ludlam, W., Kleinman, B. "The long range results of orthoptic treatment of strabismus." *Am. J. Optom. & Physiol. Opt.* 42(11):647-684, 1965.

Peters, H. B. "Vision care of children in a comprehensive health program." *J. Am. Opt. Assn.* 37(12), December 1966, updated statistics to 1979.

Selenow, A., Ciuffreda, K. "Vision function recovery during orthoptic therapy in an exotropic amblyope with high unilateral myopia." *Am. J. Optom. & Physiol. Opt.* 60(8):659-666, 1983.

Solan, H. "A rationale for the optometric treatment and management of children with learning disabilities." *J. Learning Disabilities.* 14(10), December 1981.

Solan, H., Mozlin, R., Rumpf, D. "The relationship of perceptual-motor development to learning readiness in kindergarten: A multivariate analysis." *J. Learn. Disabilities* 18(6), June/July 1985.

Vaegan: "Convergence and divergence show longer and sustained improvements after short isometric exercises." *Am. J. Optom. & Physiol. Opt.* 56(1):22-33, 1979.

Weisz, C. L. "Clinical therapy for accommodative responses: Transfer effects on performance." *J. Am. Optom. Assoc.* 50(2):209-214, 1979.

Colleges Of Optometry

(by State)

University of Alabama
School of Optometry, The Medical
Center
University Station
Birmingham, AL 35294

University of California Berkeley
School of Optometry
360 Minor Hall
Berkeley, CA 94720

Southern California College of
Optometry
2575 Yorba Linda Blvd.
Fullerton, CA 92631-1699

Illinois College of Optometry
3241 South Michigan Avenue
Chicago, IL 60616

Indiana University School of Optometry
800 East Atwater Avenue
Bloomington, IN 47401

New England College of
Optometry
424 Beacon Street
Boston, MA 02115

Ferris State College of Optometry
Big Rapids, MI 49307

University of Missouri, at
St. Louis
School of Optometry
8001 Natural Bridge Road
St. Louis, MO 63121

The Ohio State University
College of Optometry
338 West 10th Street
Columbus, OH 43210

The College of Optometry
Pacific University
2043 College Way
Forest Grove, OR 97116

Pennsylvania College of
Optometry
1200 West Godfrey Avenue
Philadelphia, PA 19141

Inter-American University of
Puerto Rico
School of Optometry
P.O. Box 3255
San Juan, PR 00936

State University of New York
State College of Optometry
122 East 25th Street
New York, NY 10010

Southern College of Optometry
1245 Madison Avenue
Memphis, TN 38104

University of Houston
College of Optometry
4901 Calhoun
Houston, TX 77004

Index

abuse, child, 183-84
Academic Therapy, 13, 183
acuity, visual, 35, 53, 56, 90, 99, 101, 104, 123, 125, 127, 160, 161,
    170, 171, 172-173
alcoholism, 5, 108, 132, 217
Alexander, E.B., 26, 27, 29, 30, 166
Altman, L.K., 39
American Academy of Optometry, 28, 262
American Optometric Association, 7, 29, 38, 41, 62,
      79-80, 81, 84, 94, 99, 143, 174, 187, 226, 230, 232, 248, 262, 273
American Optometric Foundation, 180, 181
Ames, L.B., 30, 34, 35, 272
Apell, R., 28, 67, 132, 147, 148, 235, 236
astigmatism, 5, 42, 60, 61, 65, 79-83, 84, 100, 129, 130, 233
    myopic, 83, 85, 86, 89, 91
attention deficit disorder, 123
autonomic nervous system, 91, 146

Bachara, G., 179-180, 181-183
Ballinger, B., 45
Bazin, B., 117-120, 133
bed wetting, 116
behavior, abnormal, 103, 105
behavioral optometry, (optometric vis. therapy) 2, 3, 4, 10, 15, 25, 27,
    28, 29, 35, 36, 37, 38, 42, 70, 71, 76, 77, 83, 84, 85, 86, 90, 93, 95,
    100, 102, 105, 117, 118, 138, 139, 141-142, 143, 154, 156, 157, 158,
    166, 173, 197, 215, 217, 222, 223, 226, 232, 239, 240, 244, 245,
    247, 249, 250, 251, 253, 259, 260, 261, 263, 266, 269, 270, 272, 273
Bernell Corp., 65
Bierman, A., 258-259
binocular, 24, 28, 54, 73, 134, 151, 201, 202, 204, 205, 210, 211, 250
    fusion, 56, 58, 65(?), 133
    ability, 204
binocularity, 65, 77, 88, 98, 190, 191, 203, 205, 214, 232, 236
Birnbaum, M.H., 70, 78-79, 133-134, 139
Blaise, C., 65, 183-184
blind, 97, 167, 170, 172, 209, 212, 215, 264
    cortical, 158, 159
    functional, 104
    legally, 96, 104, 209
Blouin, Jean-Paul, 150, 152
bones, 31,
    brittle, 153

Brock, F., 27, 202
Brock string, 202-204
bull fighting, 179

calcium,
    absorption, 153
    deposits, 154
Cerami, C., 149, 151, 167
Cheshire Study, 185, 186
children,
    brain injured, 27, 158
    hyperactive, 50, 123, 124
    learning disabled, 63, 102, 117-119, 159, 164, 247, 257,
        271
    vision system in, 13, 16, 31, 45, 50, 54, 60-62, 63, 68,
        73-74, 75, 76, 77, 87, 88, 104, 119, 132-133, 141-145,
        148, 158-159, 165, 171, 176, 226, 227, 234, 237, 241
Childress, C.W.*, 178-179
China, 29, 85, 158
clinics, 11, 28, 78, 185, 239, 247, 266
College of Optometrists in Vision Development, 14, 28, 29, 38, 103,
    232, 240, 259, 263, 264
Connecticut Society for the Preservation of Vision, 258, 266, 268
contacts, see lenses
convergence, 65, 67, 119, 144, 146, 147, 222
    convergence-divergence, 114, 160-161
    dynamic, 23
    overconvergence, 60
coordination, 3, 31, 47, 65, 97, 123, 141, 168, 206, 224, 229, 233, 236
    eye-hand, 12, 57, 58, 65, 66, 124, 125, 190, 228, 229, 230, 233, 234,
        237, 256
    eye-body, 121, 234
Cott, A., 63, 117, 217, 247
Crow, G., 27, 30, 31

Dallas Cowboys, 4, 173
delinquent, juvenile, 13-14, 15, 16, 18, 36, 41, 186
Dent, Bucky, 173
depression, 5, 87, 103, 105-108, 154, 217
disabled, learning, 63, 102, 117-119, 159, 164, 182, 247, 257, 271
Dowis, R.T., 16, 17
dropouts, school, 163, 183, 184
DuPont, G., 63
Driving Under the Influence (DUI), 2
Driving While Intoxicated (DWI), 2, 261-262
dyslexic, 36, 102, 120, 122, 164

Dzik, D., 16, 17

Edelman, E., 47-52, 58, 78, 97, 108-111, 116, 140, 208-215, 217-219, 271
Environmental Systems, 155
endocrine, 154
equipment, vision therapy, 65, 91, 98, 151-152, 193, 202, 270
Etting, G., 174, 175-176, 177-178
eye,
    turn, down-, in-, out-, up-, 46, 47, 56, 68, 77, 89, 95-95, 98, 130(?), 151, 160(?), 175, 189, 205-207, 209, 236, 243

farsight, see sight
Fasanella, R., 171
Feldenkrais, M., 152, 192, 193
fixation, 10, 66, 69, 70, 148, 268
Flach, F., 63, 102-103, 105, 107-108
Flax, N., 6-7, 41, 99, 140, 146, 191, 248
focusing, 12, 13, 17, 46, 56, 57, 70, 84, 88, 91, 94, 106, 107, 114, 124, 125, 127, 130, 145, 146, 147, 160-161, 202, 220, 237, 268
Forrest, E.B., 24, 27, 69, 70, 71, 72, 73, 76, 77, 78-80, 81, 197, 199-200, 227
Forkiotis, C., 1, 2-3, 53, 78, 89, 113-114, 115, 130, 131, 140, 159, 160-161, 196, 241-242, 243, 244-245, 246, 260-261, 262, 267, 271
Francke, A., 28
Friedel, D., 91, 164-166
Fulton, J., 178-179
Fuog, H., 27

Gesell, A., 27, 29-31, 32, 34, 143, 151, 269, 272
Gesell Institute
    Dept. of Vision, 31, 34, 67, 128, 166, 269
    Gesell Institute of Human Development, 27-29, 30, 35, 74, 129, 143, 159, 186, 232, 238-39, 240-241
Getman, G. N., 27, 29, 30-31, 35, 45, 156, 259, 272
Getz. D., 174, 175
golf, 176, 204

handicaps, 157, 158
Harmon, D. B., 36-37
headaches, also see migraines, 5, 9, 17, 36, 95, 108, 110, 112, 113, 114, 115, 123, 133, 147, 176, 177, 178, 179, 189, 211, 217, 218, 219, 220, 241, 245, 257, 259, 263
Hefter, T., 15
Hellerstein, L., 254, 255
holistic, 31, 139, 192

hyperopia, 65, 94

illiteracy, 41
Ilg, F., 30, 31, 34, 35, 272
Ilg, V., 31
imbalance, vision, 6, 7, 8, 9, 11, 16, 36, 38, 42, 48, 49, 56, 61-63, 67, 68, 71, 72, 75-76, 79, 82, 83, 84, 85, 86, 88-89, 91, 97-98, 102-103, 107, 110-111, 117, 121, 128, 130-133, 140-143, 145, 146-148, 151, 152, 154, 157, 163, 166, 169, 171, 176, 179, 181, 183, 193, 197, 204, 205, 214, 234, 235, 240, 241, 243-244, 267
injury,
    traumatic, 157-158
    brain, 157-158
insurance, health, 21, 39, 98, 247, 248
integration, 29, 65, 92, 123, 124, 173, 249

jaundice, 153
Johnson (Nugent), Luci Baines, 136, 137
Journal of Optometric Vision Development, 29, 69, 78, 139, 184, 264

Kane, M., 184
Kapiloff, L., 15
Kaplan, M., 102-104, 105, 107-108, 184
Kaseno, S., 12-16, 17-18, 163
Kavner, R.S., 39, 49, 63, 82, 84, 120-121, 215, 269, 272
Keystone Optical Laboratory, 155
kinesthetic, 28, 184

Lane, B., 184, 215
lens, eye, 222
lenses, 26, 37-38, 43, 85, 88, 89, 90, 91, 92, 110, 111, 112, 114, 115, 116, 119, 127, 132, 149, 150, 155, 159, 161, 167, 171, 191, 219, 220, 222-223, 224, 267
    compensating, 61, 83, 84, 86, 99, 145, 147
    contact, 10, 47-48, 113, 125, 138, 139, 177, 253
    developmental, 61, 145, 147, 148
    preventive, 145
    remedial, 89, 145
light,
    artificial, 153, 156
    and health, 152
    as nutrient, 152, 154, 156
    black, 156
    full spectrum, 152-156
    natural, 153, 154-156
    sun, 153, 154

general, 138, 250, 263
history, 28, 34, 35, 92, 166
pediatric, 65
sports vision, 28
ophthalmology, 27, 34, 38, 41-43, 46, 84-85, 142, 170
optic nerve, 6, 154, 170, 171, 173
Optometry Times, 117, 133, 146, 168
orthoptics, 20, 21, 22-23, 24, 25, 46, 77, 139
Ott, J., 155-156

Pacific University College of Optometry, 28
Padula, W.V., 158-159, 171, 265, 267, 272
palsy, spastic cerebral, 36, 158-159
parents, 29, 35, 37, 45, 49-50, 54, 60, 66-67, 71, 94, 96, 98, 104, 109,
116, 121, 123, 124, 127-128, 136, 150, 158-160, 161, 164, 167-168,
181, 187, 188, 189, 205, 206, 207, 210, 226, 229, 232, 242, 264,
266, 267, 268-269, 270
Parents Active for Vision Education, 268, 269
Peckham, E., not found -- Peckham, R.H., 27
Pepper, R., 73, 132, 184-185
perception,
depth, 58, 125, 127, 147, 175, 177-178, 179, 205, 229, 233
peripheral vision, 37, 56, 58, 104, 125, 126, 131, 171, 176, 197, 201-
202, 209, 237
Piaget, Jean, 27
pineal gland, 154
pituitary, 154
play, 5, 33, 54, 142, 148, 167, 174-175, 197, 204, 211
and visual development, 151, 177
for infants, 227-229
for toddlers, 45, 151, 152, 209, 230, 231, 234
posture, 10, 32, 73, 75, 79, 81-82, 86, 105, 116, 139, 159, 220, 225
pregnancy, 74, 75
Press, L., 23, 24, 25, 47
prism, 7, 8, 17, 22, 28, 37, 89, 122, 124, 144, 145-146, 151, 152, 172,
173, 193, 214
psychological problems, 122

Quinones, T.M., 22, 125, 127, 170-173, 258, 267

Reader's Digest, 156
reading specialist, 64, 169, 184, 206-207
Renshaw, S., 26, 53
refraction, 84, 138, 139, 252
retina, 84, 116, 141, 142, 172
Rouse, M., 15